The Hope Prescription

Mama G's Journey of Faith, Hope, and Love
Through Her Son's Childhood Cancer

GINA RASICCI RUFFA, RPh.

Foreword

In the face of life's most daunting challenges, it is often said that hope is a powerful antidote. "The Hope Prescription" by Gina Rasicci Ruffa is a poignant testament to this truth. This compelling memoir takes readers on an intimate voyage through the turbulent waters of a family's fight against cancer, not once, but twice. It is a story that resonates deeply with anyone who has faced or is currently facing similar trials.

Gina Rasicci Ruffa's narrative is anchored in the extraordinary strength of her mother, whose battle against cancer became a source of profound inspiration. This book, however, transcends a mere recounting of medical treatments and clinical experiences. Instead, it dives into the holistic and spiritual dimensions of healing, offering a comprehensive perspective on the multifaceted journey of battling a formidable illness.

"The Hope Prescription" is a rich tapestry of experiences, woven with treads of traditional medical practices, holistic healing, and the sustaining power of prayer. Ruffa eloquently illustrates how these elements intertwine to create a support system that is much about emotional and spiritual well-being as it is about physical recovery. The book underscores the essential interconnectedness of mind, body, and spirit, and presents a compelling case for a multidimensional approach to healing.

Throughout these pages, readers will find themselves immersed in the raw and authentic highs and lows of the Ruffa family's journey. The victories and the setbacks are shared with an openness that is both heart-wrenching and inspiring. The lessons learned and the resilience demonstrated serve as powerful reminders of the human spirit's capacity to endure and thrive, even in the darkest of times. Gina Rasicci Ruffa's story is just not about survival; it is about transformative power of hope and the incredible strength that can be drawn from love and unity. It highlights the profound impact that compassionate healthcare professionals can have, and the deep connections that form when people come together in the face of adversity.

"The Hope Prescription" is more than a memoir; it is a beacon of hope for anyone touched by cancer. It is a tribute to enduring human spirit and a guide for those seeking a path to healing that honors the whole person. Through her family's journey, Ruffa offers a message of resilience, love, and unwavering hope. This book is a reminder that even in our most challenging moments, the potential for profound transformation and healing is ever-present.

As you turn the pages of this remarkable book, may you find comfort, inspiration, and a renewed sense of hope. Gina Rasicci Ruffa's "The Hope Prescription" is a gift to all who seek light in the midst of darkness, and a testament to the extraordinary power of hope to guide us through life's greatest trials.

Liana Werner

– Gray bestselling author of "The Earth Diet" and "Cancer Free with Food," one of the top 100 cancer books of all time.

Dedication

I dedicate this book to my precious, strong, and selfless mother, Anita, our family matriarch. She was my biggest cheerleader, always believed in me, and inspired me to share my story. She spoke words of wisdom and taught me many valuable life lessons that have shaped me into the woman I am today. While she endured many of her own heartaches in life, she never allowed her challenges and setbacks to define her or hold her back from finding joy in every moment. For years, I watched my mom persevere and turn her cross into a crown. As the years progressed, she got better and not bitter. She held no unforgiveness in her heart. Her childlike faith, buoyant strength, and encouraging spirit made a lasting impression on every person she encountered.

I also dedicate this book to my brave son, Anthony. He is a survivor, to say the least. He has always served as a source of inspiration, courage, strength, and resilience to every member of our family. Anthony truly is the "Comeback Kid," and his enduring fortitude is one that so many people admire.

Finally, I want to thank my loving husband, Dr. Anthony Ruffa, DO, for supporting me through this journey. A special shout out to my three other amazing children, Ginelle Marie, Victor Anthony, and Giana Gabrielle, who have been my backbone, source of strength, and purpose for persevering through so many trials and tribulations.

Acknowledgement

Many thanks to my lifelong friend, Cathy, who was the first person to read through my initial draft of this story. We grew up together in West Virginia, and she knew my family personally. It must have been Divine Intervention that we became next-door neighbors in Erie, allowing her to witness many of our family's challenges as our children grew up together.

Also, a special thanks to my niece, Jennifer, who helped me edit while serving as a soundboard throughout this project.

Endless thanks to the countless prayer warriors, including friends, family, and strangers all around the country. These battle buddies and their strong intercessory prayer were paramount to Anthony's healing and recovery. All those prayers gave us **HOPE**, courage, and stamina when we felt hopeless, fearful, and weary.

About the Author

Gina Rasicci Ruffa has been a registered pharmacist for over 40 years and is nationally known for her holistic pharmaceutical skills. Gina is a cancer, health, and nutrition coach specializing in helping people obtain optimal health by *CHOICE*, not by *CHANCE*. She has worked in the pharmaceutical industry, hospital, retail, and independent pharmacy settings in several states. She is an inspiring health educator, wellness warrior, and consultant to several companies. Gina is on a mission to empower clients to *EDUCATE* before they *MEDICATE*. Gina has a strong desire to see people reach their optimal health goals, reverse disease, and live the abundant life that God has called them to live.

Gina has been interviewed on numerous podcasts and has been a radio commentator and guest speaker at several health, wellness, and cancer conferences. She is founder and CEO of What-Supp (an herbal and supplement coaching business). She assists clients in choosing natural alternatives and remedies, including herbal formulas, supplements, and plant-based foods. She advises clients on therapies that best treat their medical diagnosis' in conjunction with their pharmaceutical treatments. Gina has done extensive research on cancer prevention using natural remedies and takes an integrative approach in assisting clients to individualize which herbs, supplements, and foods would be most appropriate. She is a firm believer in lifestyle medicine and has written many health articles and blogs.

Gina is a member of NWPSHP, the Northwestern Pennsylvania Society of Health-System Pharmacists, and the FMPhA Functional Medicine Pharmacist Alliance. Mama G is widely regarded by coworkers and others as "The Plant-Based Pharmacist." As a parent of a child who battled cancer, she helps parents with the overwhelming feeling of a childhood cancer diagnosis using her **HOPE** prescriptions.

Contents

Chapter 1: Before Cancer (B.C.)

HOPE RX *"Oh, I must find rest in God only because my* ***HOPE*** *comes from Him! Only God is my rock and my salvation — my stronghold! — I will not be shaken."*

(Psalms 62:5-6)

The only time people marvel at you crying is when you come into this world. Tears are seen as an appreciation of life rather than a sign of weakness.

However, as you grow and enter new phases of life, things start to take a turn. Some roads take you to the right path, while others lead you to unexpected crossroads, which force you to journey paths that are bound to leave you with absolutely nothing. During these desolate hours of despair, we find our true strength to face the reality of our non-fiction world.

Growing up, I dreamed of living a life of happiness, starting with my loving parents, awesome siblings, and extended Italian family. I looked forward to aging with my brothers, each of us getting married, starting families, and living in good health. I even dreamed of the memories we would make as a family.

For the most part, I had a perfect childhood, complete with a textbook family and a life filled with happy times and blessings. I felt so secure in my life that I looked forward to a picture-perfect love story—being loved by a man who would be my "dream come true." My husband would share my Christian values, Italian heritage, and love for family. I thought of him as a guy who would rescue me on a white horse, just like a fairytale, and slay the demons in my life. A guy who would do anything to protect his wife and kids from the monsters lurking in the shadows, looking for a chance to prey upon the happiness of his family. But while I was dreaming up the perfect life for myself, I did not realize that dreams are called just that for a reason.

Life comes with trials, and some of us have more than others. I could wish to write my own story and have the perfect future of my dreams, but that power was not mine to hold. All I could do was go chapter by chapter, writing one word at a time to reveal the permissive will of God.

Now that I look back, flipping the pages of the chapters I've already lived through, I'm certain I would not have written my life as it played out. I realize now that everything that happened to me worked out for the better because of my relationship with Jesus.

"We know that in all things, God works for the good of those who love Him."

(Romans 8:28)

My relationship with God has helped me grow stronger spiritually through the tragedies I faced, even when they seemed insurmountable at the time. For those of you going through serious trials as I did in my life, remember this advice that was given to me:

"Understand that this too shall pass. We go THROUGH the valley of the shadow of death. We do not stay in it forever."

Despite all my years of dreaming and envisioning the perfect life, nothing prepared me for the shock that life gave me. I learned the hard way that dark times are inevitable. However, when I felt helpless and out of control, I learned to "let go and let God." I accepted that God was in complete control and I was just a passenger.

Navigating the dark times has shown me that there are few calamities no one can alter. Some of life's challenges are inescapable. But during those times, we have to learn to **HOPE** for the best and plan for the worst, trusting that God's will ultimately prevail. Everything in life is sifted through the permissive will of God, and we must be brave enough to face our trials courageously. Life is not a movie; it's an anthology of challenges written with the pen of fate. Every new story is a new chapter with an end, and every end has a new question for you to reexamine your life.

The beginning of my story takes place with the arrival of Ennio, a handsome young Italian man you'll come to know as my father. He courageously emigrated from his small hometown of Nereto, Italy (province of Teramo and region of Abruzzo) in search of a new life and exciting opportunities in the United States of America. My father had to learn the English language, which he did successfully, though he had an enduring Italian accent for the rest of his life.

His arrival in the States was nothing short of an adventure thriller. He arrived as an 18-year-old man, along with his 20-year-old sister Margaret, with very little money and no knowledge of the local language. He lived with his aunt and uncle, who helped him learn English. Despite the obstacles he faced, he became an entrepreneur and accomplished much in his life

Shortly after arriving in the States, my father met the beautiful Anita from the small town of Muse, Pennsylvania. Together, they started a family in the small steel town of Weirton, West Virginia, the Mountain State known for its breathtaking mountain views and landscapes.

. My grandmother, Adelia, was a fantastic cook and made authentic Italian cuisine from scratch. My grandfather, Alfonso, was a hard-working coal miner who loved his family dearly, especially my mother. Eventually, he passed away from black lung disease. My father's parents remained in Italy, while my mother's parents, originally from Italy, lived about an hour away from our home

Building a new life in a new town was not easy for my newlywed parents. As a young couple, they had to face a lot of challenges to build everything from nothing. My father managed to raise his children with the best resources, which required a lot of hard work and dedication. But he was determined.

My parents struggled to make ends meet. However, my siblings and I grew up with our parents' love. We were exceptionally close to each other, learning life lessons by observing our parents. They taught us the meaning and importance of a strong work ethic.

My mother was a homemaker and worked as a seamstress in our home. She was well-known for her delicious homemade bread, buns, and meatball sandwiches. One of my favorite memories with her was taking weekly trips to visit my grandmother and learning to cook at her house. My grandmother loved the kitchen and made everything with passion and authenticity.

My dad worked at Weirton Steel Mill as a foreman. He was extremely talented and smart; he designed and remodeled many apartments. He was quite proficient with his hands and also a good barber. My father had learned several trades in the Italian seminary while studying to become a priest as a young man. Priesthood did not come into play, and he left the seminary.

As a seamstress, my mom specialized in altering men's clothing and worked for a men's clothing store. She was an absolute perfectionist. Many nights, she would stay up nonstop, altering clothes. She was one of the most selfless human beings I have ever known. She looked after my grandmother, who was battling breast and colon cancer for some time. She always did so much for others but never knew how to do anything for herself.

I had two older brothers; Victor was the eldest, and David was the middle one. Being the youngest, I was pampered and coddled by both brothers. I shared a strong bond of affection and love with my extended family as well, and we often enjoyed vacations together. One of my favorite childhood memories was when my mother's parents came to visit for the holidays and filled our home with delightful food and homemade pies. When the adults got together, they often spoke Italian, and we kids would get frustrated because we did not know what they were talking about.

My grandmother loved to sing and cook, and she loved anything pertaining to health. I am pretty sure I acquired some of her genes as a health nut.

I loved my family! In fact, I think we are naturally wired to love our families and ignore their faults. I was no exception to this rule. To me, my family was faultless. They were the best people I knew in the entire world. We stood together in difficult times and celebrated each triumph together.

Our years as a family went by quickly, and before I knew it, I was attending high school with my two older brothers, who always looked out for me. Upon graduation, I decided to attend Duquesne University School of Pharmacy in Pittsburgh, Pennsylvania. I graduated in the Spring of 1983. Afterward, I moved back to West Virginia to study for my boards. I was accepted into medical school in the Fall of 1983. However, I quickly realized it was not the right fit for me, so I left after one semester.

I became an assistant manager and pharmacist for a Super X drug chain in Parkersburg, West Virginia, for nine months. In the Fall of 1984, I moved to Gainesville, Florida, where I decided to begin a one-year hospital residency program in pharmacy. After completing the program, I stayed on board and worked for the same hospital while also working on obtaining my Doctor of Pharmacy Degree. But on October 30th, 1985, everything changed.

As I was finishing my afternoon shift at the hospital, I received a phone call from my brother, Dave. In a trembling and urgent voice, he asked me to fly home as soon as possible. Something was wrong, and all I could think about was my grandmother. *Did something happen to her?*

After much persuading, Brother Dave finally disclosed the heart-wrenching news. That day, my dad and brother Victor visited my grandmother's home to help her install an electric garage opener. She was widowed at the time and needed all the extra help she could get. They were supposed to spend the night at my grandmother's house. But since it was not too late, they decided to head home instead.

On their way back to Weirton, they were struck head-on by a drunk driver driving 80 to 90 miles per hour around a blind curb. My father, brother, and the driver of the other vehicle died instantly in the violent crash. The only survivor of four was the passenger in the other vehicle.

I could not believe my ears. I did not know how to react. I remember screaming in shock and waking my roommate up. I could hardly breathe. I had a lump in my throat, and my eyes were welled with tears.

The reality was unfathomable. In no way did I want to believe what Dave was telling me. These are the kinds of stories you hear on the local news or read on the front page of a newspaper, but you never, ever expect them to happen to you or your loved ones.

I could not have even envisioned, in my worst nightmares, that my family would be the victim of such a horrific accident. The trajectory of my family's life changed forever. My brother, Victor, was only 28 years old, and my dad was also young at 52. And just like that, they were gone.

To make matters worse, Victor left behind two sons, who were 3 and 5 years old. His wife was pregnant with their third child, a precious daughter, who never got the opportunity to meet her father and experience his love. One moment of someone's recklessness and irresponsibility caused a family, *my family*, to suffer a lifetime of misery. A beautiful family was suddenly lost, cut, and severed, leaving behind many heartbroken souls in the blink of an eye.

Just a few years prior to this tragic accident, my brother Victor joined the Big Brother organization and took a young boy under his wings who had come from a single-family home. Victor was so tenderhearted toward single parents, but who would now become a Big Brother to Victor's sons to help fill the gap in lieu of his absence?

I flew back home from Florida for the funerals and to mourn our great loss. We consoled each other and tried to accept our new reality. I stayed home with my mom to help her overcome grief while battling my own. Ironically, the whole month of November was gloomy and rainy, and for many days, we lay in bed together, crying and feeling depressed. We were helpless, numb, shocked, and empty.

Grief is inevitable and painful, but you must decide whether it will make you bitter or better. God always has a purpose in our pain, and everyone deals with it differently. I did my best to help my mother, brother, and sister-in-law cope with their loss and struggle. My mother had to rise to the occasion and manage my father's apartments and rentals, becoming a landlady and bookkeeper.

I was with my family through our mourning, hoping each day we could eventually move past the grave loss we suffered. I felt sorry for my brother, who was left to fend for the entire family. Dave was only 26 years old and had such a heavy burden on his shoulders. I felt sorry for my grandmother and my widowed mother. I felt sorry for my widowed sister-in-law and for myself. My selfless brother Dave flew to Florida to help me drive a U-Haul with my belongings to move back in with my mother. No doubt, this was the longest, quietest car ride anyone could imagine. I needed to be closer to home.

I struggled through the holidays without my dad and brother and continued living with my mom. Despite our immense grief, we tried our best to cope with the situation. She encouraged me to move on with my life even though we were still reeling in shock and heartache. Like all mothers, she put herself in the backseat and placed all her focus on me. She motivated me to come out of my shell and pursue my profession.

Heavenly Father

*The death of my dear brother and father has filled my eyes with tears and my heart with sorrow. Help me to say, "Not my will, but Thine be done." Let me soon experience the healing power of my wounded heart. Teach me not to mourn as those who have no **HOPE**. Wipe away the tears from my eyes so that I may see beyond death and the grave to the resurrection and life assured by my Savior's victory over death and the grave. Let me love less the things that are material and temporal and love more the things that are spiritual and eternal. Comfort me with your consolation and have compassion on me in my suffering. May this loss be a token of Thy love. Lift me up in my distress and remind me that "All things work together for good to them that love Thee." Above all, grant me the sure conviction that Thy will and Thy ways are best so that I may emerge as a stronger Christian, better equipped to understand problems and deal with the troubles of others.*

I respected my mother's opinion about moving on with my life, and in the spring of 1986, I was finally convinced it was time to take a leap of faith and start fresh. I decided to head back to Pittsburgh because it was relatively close to my home, and I had friends there. I took a job at a local hospital as a pharmacist and attempted to put my life back together. Eventually, I started working toward new goals and opportunities. I even became an aerobics instructor—the gym was the perfect therapy for my depression. I used exercise as medicine to fight through the depression.

In 1988, at the age of 28, I met the man of my dreams—my hero. We met on a blind date arranged by one of his cousins, who was also a good friend of mine during my time at Duquesne University. The handsome guy introduced himself as Tony. He was Italian, athletic, and a medical student in Ohio. We seemed to hit it off right away. From our first date on, we understood each other, having had similar family backgrounds and spiritual values. This led us to continue dating, even though it was long-distance.

I always loved the idea of love, but my father's death served as a rude wake-up call for me. To see my mother so heartbroken and incomplete, to see her struggle to function because she lost her partner, made me think that maybe love wasn't everything. It suddenly became something I was afraid to embrace—something that I started doubting. I was afraid of losing my heart and soul like that. After losing my dad and Victor, I almost thought I had lost it all, and there was no coming back from that loss. Although three years had gone by between their passing and meeting Tony, I just knew in my heart that I was not ready to suffer like that again.

Love terrified me. I never knew if I would find a chance at love or if love would give me another chance to dwell. But Tony's appearance in my life let me break down the walls I had built around my heart. With him, I found a new purpose and persona. I could finally say that the girl from my childhood had found the hero of her dreams.

We fell in love with each other within four months of meeting, and we got engaged and married exactly on the anniversary of our first date: September 23, 1989. We were going to wait until Tony finished medical school, but we knew we were meant to be together, so we got married sooner rather than later. Our Italian families met and bonded, and our marriage ceremony was a big Italian wedding where we vowed to love each other forever. And then, a few months into our marriage, I found out I was expecting. The feeling of joy and excitement I felt erased all previous dreadful memories from my mind.

We wanted to settle down and start our own family, so once Tony completed his final year at medical school, we moved to his hometown in Erie, Pennsylvania. Tony could complete his family practice residency, and we could build a life—good things were happening.

Once Tony started his residency, I got a job as a pharmacist in the same hospital. Despite all the challenges and constraints, we worked together and saved up to buy our first house. It was a two-bedroom California-style ranch and perfect in nearly every way. The neighborhood was lovely, and we were close to a zoo and golf course. We remodeled, painted, and decorated. The changes we made transformed it from a house to a home.

I got married, acquired a new job, bought a house, and started a family—all by age 29. It was all I could ever ask for, and I was grateful for all the sudden but beautiful changes.

On October 22, 1990, my first child came into the world. He was born at the same hospital where Tony and I worked. When I heard him crying for the first time, I could only think about how melodious and euphonious it was to us. I wished I could pause that moment and replay it. He was our soft, whiny, delicate little boy. We named him Anthony Ennio after his father and my dad. The name 'Anthony' means *"priceless and praiseworthy."* Ennio means *"destined."*

As I stepped into motherhood, I felt joyous and energetic. The journey to becoming a mother was the best feeling I ever had. To feel your child growing inside your womb, coming to love that human being over nine months, and then giving birth was an unparalleled experience. Though being a new mother was highly demanding, I decided to take one step at a time and enjoy every single phase of this new life.

The bonding time you experience with your firstborn is indescribable. The infant is so dependent on their mother. Becoming a mother was one of the most satisfying and gratifying experiences of my life. The time I was able to spend with Anthony was uninterrupted and quite precious. Everyone viewed us as a perfect, happy, and successful family.

In the beginning, Tony and I needed guidance on how to handle Anthony's colic. We couldn't get the hunch, but we intuitively figured out what he wanted with time. Tony's parents, living in the same town, helped us quite a bit. My mother also made frequent trips to Erie to give us a hand as first-time parents. That was the moment I realized the story of my life was a true depiction of the word perfection. I had an amazing husband, a house, a good job, and a beautiful baby boy. The transition from a wife to a mother was indescribable in words. It felt like we had found our purpose in life.

Anthony became the center of our attention—the epitome of our lives. As I was lost in the bliss of my life, I did not realize that he had grown up into a toddler and begun to take his first steps, even though it had seemed like yesterday when I held him in my arms for the first time. It was so hard to believe that two years had quickly passed!

I remember we started having frequent excursions. As soon as Tony and I had our breaks, we both packed our bags without any hesitation and left for exciting voyages to make beautiful memories together. Tony would tell me about his childhood adventures with his dad; he wanted Anthony to have the same experiences in his life. These trips became a huge part of our lives. I used to gaze at them in awe, wondering if my story had finally found its happy ending.

We had gone on multiple trips since Anthony's arrival into our family. Tony and I explored Arizona because we enjoyed the many captivating sights. I remember how the sun-drenched desert landscape would leave us astounded. We loved it so much that we decided to come back not even a year later. We also frequently visited my mother and family in West Virginia. During these times, I realized the importance of creating family memories. When we reach the end, these are the moments we hold on to the most, cherishing the life we lived with the people we loved. Indeed, family is what keeps us alive. They are the only people with whom we can seek refuge and find protection while truly being ourselves.

While we were having the best time of our lives, Tony and I initially overlooked a few things. On vacations, we would typically see Anthony getting sick with colds and ear infections. In the beginning, we thought it was normal and did not pay too much attention to it. But over time, his illness became more frequent, and we became more vigilant and cautious.

Anthony began getting nasty ear infections and bled a lot from the left nostril. Because Tony and I were both medical professionals, we visited the pediatrician right away, who placed him on antibiotics. To avoid recurrent infections, we also had tubes placed in his ear. This method seemed effective because Anthony had a brief period of relief.

One morning, I woke up feeling nauseous and overwhelmed by my emotions. We went to see the doctor, curious and anxious to find out why this unusual morning sickness occurred. I found out I was expecting my second child. Tony and I were over the moon! It was another moment of gratitude. However, life soon took a turn, becoming challenging and much more demanding.

As Tony began to reach the end of his third year in residency, his schedule got far more hectic. He worked long shifts and had to take night calls. Little Anthony and I became particularly close. I can still see him in the back seat of my car, leaving the hospital after visiting Tony on a weekend call. Our second Christmas together was captured on videotape, and we were so excited to share it with baby Anthony.

We made the best of our time together to make as many memories as possible with our son. There was always so much that seemed to be happening all at once. Tony was busy with his schedule, and I was busy being pregnant, looking after Anthony, and catching up with work. We had a lot on our plate.

Anthony remained on antibiotics for a while, but we knew it could not be a long-term solution. Doing so usually leads to antibiotic resistance in the body, compromising the immune system and messing up the gut flora.

Being a new parent to a child, we considered it a mild sickness that would vanish with time. But one day, while I was bathing Anthony in the bathtub, I noticed the bloody noses were getting thicker and more frequent. Blood started coming out of his left nostril in copious amounts.

I was alarmed and scared. By this time, we worried that the nose bleeds and frequent ear infections were more serious than we were told. We started to doubt what we thought was normal for a toddler and rethought our decisions about our son's health. We took Anthony back to the pediatrician to express our concerns, and he referred us to a pediatric ENT (ear, nose, and throat) doctor.

With his expertise, the ENT doctor performed a nasal endoscopy and looked up Anthony's nose into his sinus area. Tony's colleagues at the hospital advised me to put my medical books away and relax. Surely, it couldn't possibly be anything too serious.

Chapter 2: Devastating Diagnosis

HOPE RX *"For I know the plans I have for you, declares the Lord, plans for welfare and not for evil, to give you a future and a **HOPE**."*

(Jeremiah 29:11)

The unpredictability of life is considered a blessing for a lot of people. They feel safe and unbothered by future events. They would rather live in the present moment, living life to the fullest. They don't believe in spending moments worrying about something they have no control over and something that is bound to happen regardless of their apprehension and anxiety.

But many people are on the other side of the table; they constantly worry about what's forthcoming in life. They can't sit back and let life happen. They want to take charge of it. Thoughts and judgments about the future naturally bind them. They can't seem to enjoy the moment they are in. They are coerced to question every decision, leading to constant nervousness and fear of the unknown.

The beauty of uncertainty is indeed unquestionable. It keeps the world moving and reminds us to stay motivated and positive. It is the only way to bring some grace in dull, dark moments of sorrow. Not only this, uncertainty is also a source of **HOPE** for a believer who submits his faith to God by believing in His countless mercies and miracles.

When I look back on the story of my life and try to compare my circumstances with the above discussion, I would not hesitate to admit the consternation that came with uncertainty. After losing the most important people to me, the major pillars of my life, to a terrible car accident, I had to start all over again with my loving husband. It amplified the importance of being uncertain yet optimistic about the future. What if Anthony's symptoms led to a discovery that we might not be able to accept? What if we encountered something that would be a source of pain and discomfort for our precious son?

The winter of 1993 was dreary. It was a time when the sky was overcast with clouds, and the chilly winds blew everywhere. The temperature almost went down to minus degrees. It also began to snow heavily, which made everything look dull, foggy, and dreary.

Anthony loved playing in the snow. He was mesmerized by the snowflakes twirling right from the sky. He loved how beautifully everything got covered up with a white blanket. He and I used to make snowballs and drop them over each other. But then his symptoms started becoming more severe, and we agreed to consult the ENT specialist, as I mentioned previously.

We were concerned about his health more than any other thing in the world. However, we were somewhat fearful regarding the findings. At that crucial time, I needed someone to be on my side besides Tony. I informed my mom and my brother Dave about Anthony's non-resolving condition and how it kept getting worse. I felt deeply broken and shattered by everything that was happening, but my mother reminded me,

*"This is how God tests the people He loves, and we should not lose **HOPE** in his mercy."*

After realizing the intensity of my situation, my brother and mother immediately packed up their things and left for Erie. When we were finally in the exam room, I realized we might leave the room as different people. Our lives might change forever by whatever news we would get from Anthony's doctor.

As the doctor noticed our concern for Anthony's condition, he reassured us by stating that it was most likely nothing too serious. It was what we had been wanting to hear. After thoroughly discussing Anthony's medical history and the nasal endoscopy that revealed some hindrances in his way, the doctor repeated the process just to be sure. Then, he advised us to get a C.T. scan to rule out anything critical.

The doctor seemed perplexed by the reports after the scan was performed. He detected an abnormal mass in one of Anthony's sinuses. Afterward, a follow-up MRI was advised to confirm the finding. We waited hours to verify if the previous diagnosis was correct or just a misunderstanding.

One test after another kept piling up the emotions I was holding onto. I wanted to stop all of this. I regretted showing up at the hospital. I could not stand my son going through all those tests. He was a tiny, innocent boy who dreamt of growing old with his friends and family like any other child. He was such a trooper, yet it was difficult for him to understand what was happening at such an early age. He watched Donut Man videos and Veggie Tale videos about Jesus.

I kept all these sentiments aside and focused merely on his diagnosis. I wished I could swipe those terrible moments from my sight, but it was the time to stay strong for my son.

The doctor finally called us into the room again and confirmed the presence of a mass through the MRI reports. I thought he was disclosing that intense revelation to someone else. The doctor reiterated the statement to make us realize the seriousness of this situation.

To further rule out the intensity of the mass, he advised us to go for a biopsy. As soon as he uttered that word, I began to tremble. Tony draped his arms around me and gave me a tight hug. He reminded me to stay calm because my body wouldn't be able to tolerate the shock, especially with another life inside of me, my second child.

It was hard for both of us to accept or imagine the news. Tony got through that period by distracting himself with work. I was on a mission to dedicate my life to caring for Anthony through this ordeal.

I could not think of anything else except my son's health. I picked out every book I knew and searched nearly every article about his condition. I even considered any tiny bit of information that would make my son's health better. I related to the father in the movie *Lorenzo's Oil,* who would go to the ends of the earth to try to find a cure for his son. I was suddenly on a mission to exhaust every possible option to help my child.

I felt a huge responsibility on my shoulders to find the right solution for my son's condition. While I was busy doing all the research, the medical professionals discouraged me from investigating this and dismissed it as benign inflammatory polyps.

As Tony was doing his residency at the same hospital, he was acquainted with all the medical staff and workers. Some of his colleagues assured him that the mass was likely a benign lesion. Others suggested it to be inflammatory polyps. Either way, it was predicted to be harmless. That made us confident that things were still in our favor and that the biopsy would rule out all the doubts we had been enduring in our minds.

After much conversation, Tony and I gave a green signal for the biopsy. I was eagerly waiting for the doctors to assure me it was a benign mass and there was nothing to worry about.

Watching my son, a little boy, experience the rough side of life so early was not easy. My soul wanted to leave my body before I witnessed any of this. But I had to be strong for Anthony and the baby inside my womb.

The moment was profound. All these medical professionals around him were preparing for a biopsy, and he was looking outside at the snow where any young child would prefer to be, *should* be, but he was unable to play.

As Anthony entered the operating room, I stepped back from the hall. I wished I could stand beside him, but he had to take this path alone. The biopsy was supposed to be quick, so I decided to stand next to the door to make it to Anthony as soon as he was done. I kept waiting, but he did not come out.

During the delay, I prayed and stared out the window. The snow had not stopped, and it started to change into a storm. The visibility was very poor, making it seem almost impossible to go back home.

Instead of being over quickly, what was supposed to be a short biopsy turned into a three-and-a-half-hour surgery. With every passing moment, my heart felt like it was skipping beats. Finally, we learned the doctors were successful in taking out the samples from the mass for the purpose of diagnosis.

During the surgery, the doctors sent the frozen preliminary samples to the laboratory for histological examination. Before Anthony came out of the operating room, we were informed by the doctor the mass was benign. It was a moment of relief for all of us. Those were the exact words we were praying to hear.

Throughout this whole ordeal, my mom and Dave stood with me, acting as my rock. It was my brother Dave's birthday and family circumstances had to pull Dave away early, but my mom stayed by my side until Anthony fully recovered.

Due to heavy storms, the city was camouflaged in a white layer of snow. We decided to spend that night at the hospital as Anthony rested. After a long fight with the snow, the sun's rays finally crossed through the window. The next morning was bright and sunny, and we wanted to take our son home as soon as possible.

While Anthony was in the hospital room, two doctors came in; one of them was a pathologist. They were carrying final biopsy reports in their hands, and the expressions on their faces were somber.

During my years of experience in the medical profession, I have never seen a pathologist deliver pleasant news to anyone. They are believed to carry loads of awful news. My intuition was not wrong. On March 13th, 1993, the pathologist informed us that the mass, which initially appeared to be merely a benign lesion, was, in fact, a poorly differentiated tumor, which means it did not have a good prognosis.

"What did you say, a tumor? A poorly differentiated tumor?" I stuttered.

We were foolish enough to think it was a benign mass that would resolve over time. We were naïve enough to think it would go away like in any other normal child. Now, they exploded this news like a missile without any warning.

Tony grabbed a water pitcher from the table and threw it onto the floor. He had been calm and composed throughout the whole ordeal, but having his worst fears confirmed was too much for him.

The thing that really disturbed him was that the hero couldn't save his family. While we both were crying and questioning our lives, we decided to hold on and keep faith in God. We informed our fellow church members about the dreadful discovery of Anthony's diagnosis.

They all came to the hospital right away, concerned about Anthony's health. With loving arms, they embraced and consoled us while intently praying for Anthony. Over the next week, we processed denial, anger, grief, shock, and fear.

"I must express my anguish. My bitter soul must complain."

(Job 7:11)

The senior pastor at our church had a close bond with Anthony. He came to the hospital to support and counsel us as we badly needed it. His spiritual perspective about these tough times gave us a new ray of light. He encouraged our faith and provided us with new **HOPE**. Through his talk, we began to think positively despite the despair overtaking us. He asked us to submit our matter to God and confide in him. He quoted **(Psalm 91:2-4):**

"He that dwelleth in the secret place of the Most High shall abide under the shadow of the Almighty. I will say of the Lord; He is my refuge and my fortress; my God, in Him will I trust."

Those verses provided us with a sense of relief amid chaos. As soon as the pastor left, Tony and I wanted to clear our minds with the trauma and restart the process all over again. We didn't want to disclose any of this to our little boy. So, we headed toward home to process all the events that happened that day and think with clear heads.

We couldn't leave Anthony alone at the hospital, so my mom decided to stay with him. Although the sun had shown its light, the previous night's snowstorm was extreme enough to cause trouble on the way home.

The snow reached up past our knees, and we were left with the option to walk since our car was stuck in a snow drift. Tony left the car on a boulevard, and we covered the distance on foot. My body had already been pushed beyond its strength, and I was walking home in knee-deep snow, nine months pregnant and exhausted. As I stumbled my way forward, I started to think back on my life since losing the two most important people: my dad and eldest brother, Victor. Their loss was enough to break my heart into pieces. I was left with no confidence in love or friendship. But then Tony came along and changed that for me.

He gathered all the broken pieces and glued them back together. He made me believe in my story again and made me live in the world of my fantasy. He became the hero of my nearly broken life.

Since meeting him, I felt better. I felt happier than I ever did. Every day in my married life was full of achievements in terms of being a wife, a mother, and a pharmacist. But fate intervened with Anthony's diagnosis.

Now, it seemed like everything had stopped. I could sense a force pulling me back into the black hole. I felt so powerless. I couldn't escape it. I didn't want to think of losing my son as I had lost my dad and Victor. These thoughts haunted me as much as I tried to distract my mind.

The circumstances were too much to digest. I was 38 weeks pregnant, and Tony was about to finish his residency in the next three months. We were supposed to celebrate these moments of happiness together. We were so close to the idea of a perfect family.

Instead of being happy, we were mourning the heart-wrenching discovery of our son's cancer diagnosis. This unexpected route that life chose for us brought so many questions that I had difficulty comprehending. What wrong have we done in life? Why was it happening to us? Why were we the victims of this misfortune? How would we survive this? These questions pooled up in our minds, but we couldn't find any reasonable answer to satisfy ourselves. Anthony was our first-born child. He was the source of joy and happiness in our lives. My life was nearly complete to perfection. I had a loving husband with a cute, tiny boy, and in a few weeks, I was about to bring a new life into this world.

A part of us still wondered if the cancer diagnosis was just a bad dream. Sadly, it was not.

The doctors suggested a few options for Anthony's treatment, but they were challenging and very risky. According to them, this form of cancer was rare and virulent in children, with only a 50% chance of survival.

As a pharmacist married to a physician, we never thought handling this life-threatening disease would be so overwhelming and devastating.

We wanted a second opinion to reconfirm the diagnosis. We had questions and reservations regarding the treatment options. So, after breathing deeply, we decided to stay optimistic about our son's future. We were determined to go till the very end of the road to seek better treatment for Anthony if needed.

Previously, we had spent the holidays in multiple places. But that year was different. Instead, we were not traveling for enjoyment but to explore the alternatives for our delicate little boy.

To confirm the diagnosis of cancer, we headed to Children's Hospital in Pittsburgh. Testing started with a myriad of C.T. scans, MRIs, spinal taps, bone marrow biopsies, and blood tests. There was so much blood that was drawn from my little son's veins, and he quickly became a pin cushion with frequent pricks and pokes. My heart broke for the innocence he was losing as a toddler.

I remember gazing at the nurse pricking my boy and imagining the pain he must have been going through. We wished so hard to take his place on the bed. We felt horrible about every single poke and needle prick. Tony held him tight as he was in pain, and Anthony kept saying, *"Daddy hurt! Daddy, help me*!!" We wanted to bear all his suffering, but all we could do was stand there and watch, helpless to save him from this torment. It was the hardest thing we ever had to do.

The test results came in, and we met with the pediatric oncologist. He sat us down and confirmed the presence of a Stage 3 cancer called Rhabdomyosarcoma (RMS). The doctors in Pittsburgh seemed disappointed that we did an actual surgery in Erie rather than just performing the biopsy.

The doctors believed the mass, being close to the pituitary gland, was too large to perform surgery. They encouraged chemotherapy to shrink it for a more successful surgical outcome and offered us three options. We were forced to decide quickly to get the tumor under control.

Tony and I were at an impasse. We wanted what was best for our son. But we also knew of the potential side effects chemotherapy could cause, especially while his brain was still developing.

Would Anthony become sterile? Would he have facial asymmetry after radiation? Would radiation stunt his growth and affect his brain since the tumor was close to his pituitary? Would the high doses of chemotherapy make him susceptible to cancer recurrence? All these questions were thrown at the oncologist one after the other. We couldn't figure it out, though we were medical professionals. We had to choose between the gold-standard protocol and some experimental ones.

Our oncologist counseled us to treat the cancer first without predicting the side effects it would bring later. We knew every treatment would have consequences, so starting as early as possible was better. Therefore, we chose to stick to the gold-standard chemotherapy for RMS. It became our first step toward searching for the latest Rhabdomyosarcoma (RMS) treatment worldwide.

How would we ever make this *mess* into a *message*? Only by God's grace and power. If He brought us *to* this, He would get us *through* this.

We faced many tear-filled sleepless nights. Sometimes, the waves come crashing at us. But we tried hard to remember this: "The bumps are what we climb on."

But why so many bumps in my life? Was this to make me stronger? We have choices and can either turn to *despair* or *dependence* on God.

We chose to depend on God. After all, we had to fight the good fight with all our might for our precious little son. We prayed beautifully with Anthony every single night, pointing to his tumor and saying, "Go away, Jesus, heal me."

Chapter 3: Homecoming Homework

HOPE RX *"But in your hearts revere Christ as Lord. Always be prepared to give an answer to everyone who asks you to give the reason for the **HOPE** that you have. But do this with gentleness and respect."*

(1 Peter 3:15)

There is no doubt in the mercy of God. His plans always find a way that we fail to acknowledge. He makes a way when there seems to be no way.

Indeed, darkness offers the realization of His existence. It gives us a moment to close our eyes and comprehend His presence. Not only that, but it helps to build a ray of **HOPE** that flashes light from an unexpected source.

The leap of faith has held up my whole life. Throughout my journey, I gripped the ropes tight each time to prove my resilience and strength. I am not afraid to admit the inconvenience it brings, but I always believed in the power of prayer. It feels such a relief to submit the worries in front of the Lord in the **HOPE** and assurance that His promises are true.

After my son's distressing diagnosis of cancer, I asked myself two questions.

Would you complain about the circumstances that God has put you in?

Or would you try to find a solution to this problem?

I was the person who would choose the latter. I recalled all the significant events that almost broke me, but I stood up every time stronger than before. It looked almost like the end of the world. But later, I realized the motives behind those hurdles—every hardship uplifted my faith instead of shattering it.

Everything in life gets sifted through the permissive will of God, remember? Then, who are we to question our Lord, the creator of the universe?

Ever since I was a little girl, I had an inquisitive nature. I was naturally curious, and I wanted to know everything about everything. I would open books to gather every ounce of knowledge. However, I regret never paying attention to this capability as a gift until I needed it the most.

After the confirmation of cancer by the pediatric oncologist, Tony and I had to choose the right treatment plan for our son. Though we were aware of the condition, we never thought we would have to deal with it this intimately.

I became entirely consumed with research because I was a researcher by nature. We had to look at this obstacle as an opportunity to take advantage of my gift from God.

Anthony had RMS (Rhabdomyosarcoma), which is a rare and virulent cancer. This soft tissue sarcoma usually begins in the muscles attached to bone, and it can metastasize to other areas of the body. This cancer most often spreads to the lungs, lymph nodes, and bones.

The etiology behind this diagnosis is mainly unknown. I read that each year, about 400-500 people are diagnosed with RMS, most being children or teens. The majority of children suffering from RMS are younger than ten years old, and it is more common in boys. There are four stages: Stages I and II do not have evidence of spread to lymph nodes or distant sites. Stage III has local lymph node involvement, and Stage IV spreads to distant nodes and sites. Stage IV has the lowest survival rate.

After understanding this condition, I began exploring all the possibilities to help make Anthony better. My research began with Complementary Alternative Medicine (CAM), including supplements, juicing, smoothies, and natural remedies. I dove deep into integrative and alternative therapies to maximize Anthony's chance of survival. I didn't limit myself to one solution; instead, I looked at any regime that could improve his prognosis. But, I always had to weigh the potential benefit vs. the potential risk. We were suddenly running a marathon we had not trained for—we had no idea how long and intense it would be, nor the duration. But gaining the stamina we needed to run this intense race was an absolute necessity.

I also approached every pediatric oncology center in the country, consulting with healthcare professionals to discern the best possible outcome for Anthony's condition. We were trying to determine the best options for our two-year-old son. It is not valid to impose standard treatment for every person; each individual's needs differ. Therefore, as parents and healthcare professionals, we knew experimental and established protocols were already in place.

After considering these experimental protocols with little evidence and study to provide enough satisfaction, Tony and I felt more solace in initiating the gold-standard protocol therapy, which had a 50/50 chance of remission and survival rate. This protocol therapy maximized Anthony's time at home, minimizing his time in the hospital, which would be more manageable for all of us.

Choosing what to do for our little one was probably the hardest decision ever to make! No parent ever wants to be in the place where Tony and I were. Determining the fate of our child was severely painful.

As parents, it felt like a massive burden. We wanted the most effective and least painful pathway since Anthony was too young to make those decisions for his life. We wanted to cover all our fundamentals so we could look back and say we did everything conceivable to maximize the chance of Anthony's long-term survival.

Amid the chaos, it almost felt like Tony and I were on a seesaw. Whoever was up had to encourage the one who was down.

Finally, the day arrived; it was the first round of Anthony's chemotherapy. Tony and I had mixed feelings. A part of us was content with the decision we made; the other part had doubts and fear. Regardless of the roller coaster of emotions, we put our complete faith in God and prayed for

Anthony's well-being and a good response with minimal side effects.

We took Anthony to Children's Hospital in Pittsburgh with many expectations, along with faith and **HOPE** to return home soon. We stayed at the Ronald McDonald House (RMH) to rest in between our long days at the hospital. Meanwhile, Anthony got his Mediport catheter inserted to begin the chemotherapy. We stayed with him as much as possible to console him. But God's plans are indeed better than ours. His techniques are merely the definition of perfection. All these engagements made me forget about my pregnancy because Tony and I were fully focused on Anthony's health.

Before I could go to the hospital with my son, I went into labor at the Ronald McDonald House. It was a surprise because it happened 15 days before my due date. Perhaps it was all the stress and anxiety that made it happen sooner than expected.

Instead of rushing to the hospital for the delivery, I went to Children's Hospital to be at Anthony's side.

There, it became apparent to the staff that I was in full-blown labor. They insisted I go to the women's hospital to have the baby delivered, but I was so reluctant to leave Anthony alone at the oncology unit.

It was Anthony's first round of chemotherapy, and I wanted to be there for him. I was suffering with critical contractions that made me want to scream out loud, but I didn't want to make it apparent to the staff. I knew my pain was less than Anthony's, so I decided to endure quietly. However, the staff eventually refused to let me stay and transferred me to Magee Women's Hospital.

I had experienced most of the labor alone, refusing to leave Anthony. So, within a half hour of the arrival at the hospital, our newborn baby came into the world. I remember the staff attempting to start me on IV fluids, but the birthing occurred so quickly that they forgot to hook me up, and blood from my arm spilled all over the floor.

Right after the doctors delivered the baby, I could see their happy faces saying, "Congratulations, Gina! Your baby is healthy and beautiful!"

I was thankful to God for His blessings. I asked the doctor, "Is it a boy or a girl?"

The doctor replied with joy, "Gina, it's a girl!"

When Tony and I heard those words, my heart swelled with all the happiness I could feel. All the negative thoughts vanished from our heads. We took it as a sign from God that Anthony would be able to grow up with his little sister.

Our daughter's birth was a moment of relief and liberation from the feelings I'd been holding on to for quite a while. The truth is, as soon as I had found out about my pregnancy, I had a fear of having a boy who might serve as a replacement for Anthony, just in case anything happened to him. God gave me a *Rhema* word from (**Psalm 118:17**):

"I shall not die, but live, and declare the works of the Lord."

I had forgotten the kindness behind God's actions. When I heard about the baby girl, I took it as a symbol for Anthony's long life from God's will.

*"Now faith is confidence in what we **HOPE** for and assurance about what we do not see."*

(Hebrews 11:1)

When I held the baby, I was in awe. She was a cute little newborn, crying gently in my arms as I smiled back at her. Tony and I named her Ginelle Marie, which means *"God is gracious"* and *"wished for child."*

Tony and I tirelessly managed things together. We would walk up and down the hospital's halls to ensure everything was in order. We often questioned each other, "What the heck is going on? How and why did this happen?" Thankfully, we also had family beside us. My mother and sister-in-law were there, providing me with comfort and support.

Knowing that two different people from the same family were at separate hospitals was surreal. Both were seeking treatment, but one life was dependent on it while the other just birthed a new life into the world. Our son was at Children's Hospital receiving his chemotherapy while I was at Magee Women's Hospital delivering his little sister.

Though thrilled with the newborn life, we were also uncertain of the future of our firstborn. Anthony and I were released from our respective hospitals on the same day and returned to Erie.

The circumstances were overwhelming for us both. We just had a newborn baby who was so loveable. And Anthony had made it through his first round of chemotherapy. We didn't know what to expect.

I kept my bags packed for Children's Hospital, two hours away from our home, in case Anthony experienced fever or sickness in between rounds of harsh induction chemotherapy. We remained vigilant and prepared for anything that might come up.

Anthony's chemotherapy rounds were three weeks apart, and he had to receive daily Neupogen shots to help his white blood cells recover in time for the next round of chemo.

My boy was such a trooper through the innumerable spinal taps, CT scans, MRIs, bone scans, port placements, needle jabs, and injections. You name it, he received it. We were so afraid of the long-term side effects, but we had no choice but to walk by faith in the **HOPE** of a cure. We always surrounded him with Power Rangers, telling him they would kill the bad guys (the cancer cells). He used to relate to that story, which helped him psychologically.

It felt like we had restarted our family. Ginelle brought a new sense of **HOPE** in these difficult times, and seeing our children together was lovely. I could finally witness many beautiful memories and moments between the siblings.

Yet the hard times carried on. Once, during a chemotherapy session, I fell ill and couldn't be at the hospital with Anthony. I was not going to expose him to my sickness. Meanwhile, Tony was busy with his demanding residency schedule. Fortunately, my in-laws offered to travel to look after their grandson on our behalf. Anthony's fever and low white blood cell count (WBC) required him to stay in the hospital for ten consecutive days.

Staying away from my child was not easy, as he always needed me by his side. When he returned home, my eyes filled with tears just from hearing his voice. He stumbled into the house, appearing like a malnourished child from a third-world country, but still retained his resiliency.

With clumps of hair falling out, he ran toward me. I could not believe the hasty changes that had occurred in such a short period. Anthony had become so weak and thin because of his nausea and small appetite. It was hard for him to keep anything down. He used to say in his cute little voice, *"Mommy, don't be sad. Me sad, too."*

His treatment became part of our routine. We started to adapt to the schedule with frequent commutes to Pittsburgh. Most of the time, we had to stay at the hospital for a few days. It usually took a couple of days to make sure his kidneys were protected and well-hydrated before administering the chemotherapy. We prayed day and night for the chemotherapy to debulk the tumor so that surgery had a higher chance of success. We would pray as a family to take Anthony's cancer, fever, tummy aches, sore throats, and mouth sores away. Anthony would point to his tumor and say his constant prayer, "Go away! Jesus, heal me."

After several rounds of chemotherapy and hospitalizations for fever, neutropenia, and infections, which could all have been fatal, we made it through the first stage.

I never thought I would be strong enough to bear all of this. Sometimes, worrying about things I have no control over feels so pointless. However, at that time, it felt like the end of the world. Tony and I didn't give up on our son's health for a second. We made sure everything was being done correctly despite all that was happening. I was the crazy pharmacist mother who appeared in the med room with my calculator to check and double-check each dose of chemotherapy that my precious son was to receive.

For four months, Anthony's treatments took place without any breach. We were determined to hear good results from the treatment. The doctors conducted some tests to evaluate the mass. The results were satisfying.

Finally, some good news!

We found out that Anthony's tumor responded to the chemotherapy. The size of the mass was reduced by 65%, which was a milestone. Tony and I were happy with the report. It gave us **HOPE** that our son would come out of this misery after all.

The next step was the most crucial of all the choices we made. Despite our experiences and knowledge in the field, we both were trembling while thinking about heading on to radiation and possible skull-based surgery. During our stay in Pittsburgh, we managed to get an appointment with a reputable surgeon. He seemed satisfied with the chemotherapy and gave us the green signal to proceed with the surgery. However, he also mentioned a postoperative complication that built some reservations in our minds.

The doctor told us, "A consequence of the surgery would be the loss of his sense of smell." Just picturing our little boy losing one of his special senses at this stage crumbled our souls. Therefore, we persevered to find an option that would not let him lose this critical sense.

Tony and I had only one question: *What if?*

Though it was not wise to stray from the situation, we could not control our thoughts. We called every national cancer institute worldwide to find the best surgeons, including ones in Switzerland, Italy, Colorado, Vancouver, and countless others.

I remember spending hours researching and studying to find the best treatment for his diagnosis. I accumulated substantial phone bills and filled numerous notebooks with information gathered during these calls.

After multiple attempts and with the help of God, we finally found the right doctor, Dr. Victor. Originally from Pittsburgh, he was a skull-based surgeon practicing in

Denver. We discussed our concerns and doubts about the surgery with him, including the potential loss of smell.

Dr. Victor assured us that his approach would spare Anthony's sense of smell. He was confident in his method and believed he could make it happen. It wouldn't be wrong to say that he was a true blessing. Tony and I were satisfied with him and decided to head to Denver. We packed for this unexpected adventure, feeling optimistic and hopeful. We were determined to make this work at any cost.

Before leaving Pittsburgh, I sought all the prayers and blessings from the people around us. I mailed out detailed newsletters to friends, family, and church groups with precise directions to pray for Anthony's life. The letter contained details about all the upcoming procedures, risks, side effects, and potential problems that might arise.

With the positive results of Anthony's chemotherapy and the birth of Ginelle, I started to recover from my past traumas. But it was God's guidance. Even during this challenging time, He showered His blessings upon my family and me.

When I look back on the moment that I found out about Anthony's diagnosis to the time I was mentally preparing for his surgery, there's a vast transformation in my personality. I was lost in despair and questioned every single decision I had made in my life. But then, with the help of God and enough grace and strength that He provided me, I became steadfast. If a parent can watch their angel go through this, they can take on any calamity that might appear later. When

I first became a mother, I never thought, in my wildest dreams, I would have to witness this type of suffering. I had no idea how painful it can be to see your young child endure such hardships. We had a choice of being paralyzed in fear or pressing through the fear. We chose the latter.

"I can do all things through Christ which strengthens me."

(Philippians 4:13)

I began to believe in my story again. *God will somehow turn this TRIAL into a TRIUMPH and this TEST into a TESTIMONY someday.* I witnessed my hero, Tony, trying so hard to protect his family from all the evils but ultimately leaving all matters into God's capable hands. It is all about timing and God's Master Plan. Only the Great Physician can change the dimension of life from impossible to possible.

"With man, this is impossible, but with God, all things are possible."

(Matthew 19:26)

While at Children's Hospital, Tony and I bonded closely with another family from Erie, the Edingers. Christy and Mike's son, little Mikie, had AML (acute myeloid leukemia). They had arrived at Children's Hospital in Pittsburgh the same month we did, March 1993. Mikie battled leukemia for 18 months before losing his fight on July 8, 1994. He was only three years old. He had undergone numerous rounds of chemo and radiation along with two bone marrow transplants, one using his marrow and the other using a matched unrelated donor from Germany. Christy and

I were both pregnant with our daughters that year. We used to walk up and down the hospital aisles with our IV poles and sons, wondering how we both ended up on the pediatric oncology unit—a parent's nightmare. Tony and I often felt so bad that our son was making it through his battle, but their son had lost his. It just didn't seem right or fair.

"It is better to trust in the Lord than to put confidence in man. It is better to trust in the Lord than to put confidence in princes."

(Psalms 118:8-9)

Chapter 4: Saving Surgery

***HOPE Rx** "Why, my soul, are you downcast? Why so disturbed within me? Put your **HOPE** in God, for I will yet praise Him, my Savior and my God."*

(Psalm 42:11)

Life is like a roll of dice. You have yet to determine what the next throw will bring. The numbers on the dice decide the fate of the player. Sometimes, even the good numbers make you lose, and wrong numbers let you win.

In the end, it's all in the hands of fate. You may not have a say in the matter.

The dice of my life rolled in directions I never comprehended. Some decisions were in my control, while others were out of my hands. The silver lining of all the hurdles in my life is that I never cheated; I always played my part with honest intentions.

God has always been on my side because of the transparency in my soul. He knew my heart was compassionate, and I could never harm someone's life, even for a moment. God chooses people to assess their patience in difficult times and rewards them accordingly. I am not afraid to say He chose me.

After receiving the good news of Anthony's tumor regression, we were a bit stress-free for a while. I had a rough time during his chemotherapy and giving birth to baby

Ginelle. But Tony's support got me through it all. We had a lot to handle at once, but we did it! We survived with the help of many peoples' consistent prayers and faith in God, which helped us reach the next step toward saving our little son's life.

Together, we discussed our doubts about the surgery, which kept us awake the night before the scheduled date. However, the surgeon was adamant about the best possible outcomes the procedure would bring. We were content with what Dr. Victor had in mind for Anthony's recovery and decided to head to Denver.

Tony and I have always been fond of traveling. We wanted to go everywhere possible in the world. We always had a desire to explore and discover new sites and places. Little did we know that our craving would cost us a considerable price financially and emotionally.

I started packing with all the necessary stuff that came into my mind. And I packed something for myself or perhaps my soul—**HOPE**, lots of it. I intended to return home again with pleasure, leaving behind all the misery and sorrow back in Denver.

In early June 1993, my family arrived at the airport to depart for Denver. While we were waiting, a Christian man who worked for Compassion International sat next to us. I looked frightened, with stress lines on my forehead. He noticed my suffering and asked, "Hi, what's wrong? Is everything alright?"

The moment he showed his concern, I burst into tears. I couldn't resist. I told him my story and about why we were heading to Colorado. He consoled me with all his virtues and persuaded me to stay focused on Anthony. He was wearing a baseball cap that caught my sight; it said, "God's side."

He took it off his head and handed it to me for Anthony. Holding it in my hand, I felt God was answering my questions. It gave me a sense of relief that God had taken matters into His hands and would look after all of my family. The cap was a sign that God *really* was on our side.

Though we may not recognize or feel God's presence, the truth is He is always there, strengthening and empowering us. Though we may not believe it, in actuality, He provides power so that the ordeals do not destroy us in any way.

After landing safely in Denver, we spent the first night at a Ramada Inn. Tony and I were skeptical about the surgery. But, no matter how difficult and painful this process was, we kept encouraging each other to build enough resilience.

"We have to be strong for our son and daughter." We said this to each other while looking into each other's eyes, holding hands firmly.

We were finally at a stage where Anthony became a candidate for surgery. He was unbelievably courageous. He became my little hero through it all with such stamina and strength.

Looking back on the process, I would never have imagined how strong I was until it all happened. I was finally and reluctantly embracing the surgery—but the reality was shaking me inside out. Everything was happening so fast. Anthony had a life-dependent surgery in a few days, baby Ginelle was now three months old, and Tony had just completed his residency requirements. He missed his graduation ceremony in Pennsylvania and spent it at the Ronald McDonald House (RMH) instead. So many emotions gathered up!

Tony will never forget how he used to walk down the street, carrying Anthony on his shoulders and wondering: How could a small boy be so skinny and weak?

Tony's parents were supportive, and they had a special bond with Anthony. They were willing to play their part, so we flew them to Denver to help us. The scenes were quite upsetting at the RMH. It seemed as though one child was sicker than the other. It was depressing to watch other families go through the same as we were, but it also consoled us that we were not alone in our journey.

I used to think that God was testing my faith only. But when I saw other families at the Ronald McDonald House suffering just as badly, I couldn't resist being grateful to Him for His mercy and kindness.

Our daily routine at the RMH was far from ordinary, full of tasks and errands. The pattern consisted of Anthony's IV therapy sessions, home health nurse visits, and pediatric oncology appointments. We even had a special photography session to take pictures to remember this time. It was surreal and soothing at the same time. Yet I couldn't help but think: *Who would want to remember this time?*

During our stay, Tony and I would take our kids to the city park—we longed for normalcy and distraction. We met so many families there who were in the same shoes as us. Specifically, I remember one exceptional family from Montana whose 15-year-old son, Doug, had been battling a brain tumor. Doug was like a big buddy to Anthony and shared a fond affection toward him.

An Assembly of God church also prayed over Anthony, and Tony spent much time studying for his boards. Fortunately, he was able to schedule his testing in Denver. As we reflected on Anthony's surgery, God allowed Tony to take his boards beforehand, which was a blessing in disguise.

While everything was happening, Tony and I didn't stray from our purpose of visiting Denver. We scheduled an appointment with Dr. Victor, who explained all the potential things that could go wrong with surgery. Specifically, he mentioned:

"Anthony would have to get a tracheostomy prophylactically so that his airway would not cut off with all the head swelling that would occur postoperatively."

Hearing these words almost made me want to fly home out of fear. Yet Tony and I had been mindful of every risk and medical mountain that could ascend with such a severe procedure. So, we had Dr. Victor schedule the surgery for the morning of June 23.

I didn't know what to feel or think. I was anxious about the forthcoming, but I was glad we would leave all this chaos behind and finally begin our average happy family life. Tony and I didn't let go of each other during that difficult time. We were perplexed but decided to submit our faith in God and had complete confidence in His mercy.

"What I feared has come upon me; What I dreaded has happened to me. I have no peace, no quietness; I have no rest, but only turmoil."

(Job 3:25-26)

Although we had finally decided on the surgery, God's plan was remarkable and unquestionable. He had a different plan for our baby, which was better.

It was dark at midnight when it happened. I couldn't sleep because I kept thinking about the surgery. I was partly awake and wanted to take another glance at my son before the procedure. Suddenly, I noticed a strange change in Anthony's condition. He became febrile with a high-grade fever, which seemed like a threat to break all our **HOPES**.

Tony and I didn't expect that change of events at the point when we were finally ready to go on with the surgery. We were so worried by his condition that we literally ran toward the hospital.

At 4 AM, we entered the emergency room. Anthony's temperature kept rising as his blood pressure dropped. He went into septic shock, which is considered a severe, potentially life-threatening infection and must be treated emergently before any procedure. Another mountain threatened to crush our **HOPES**.

The hospital admitted Anthony immediately and postponed his pre-planned surgery. Later, the doctors placed him on outpatient intravenous antibiotic therapy, which continued at the RMH for two weeks.

This is how life happens. It doesn't go as planned. Perhaps the uncertainty is a blessing; in my case, it was. Regardless, some thoughts did leave my mind. There was a war going on between my head and heart. I kept thinking: Would Anthony be lost before our family could even try for his best chance at life?

Holding on to the emotions that kept piling up was difficult. Psyching oneself up for such suffering is no easy matter. The postponement caused us additional emotional havoc because we worried the cancer would grow since we had to reschedule the surgery and postpone chemotherapy.

With each fever came multiple needle sticks, blood draws, spinal taps, chest X-rays, and CT scans. Instead of spending two weeks in Denver, we spent over a month there.

Anthony became fragile with each passing day, and his immune system was compromised. He needed a break and wanted to go out and play like a regular toddler. He wanted to run without gasping for air like an older man.

At last, the day came that we had been waiting for impatiently. On July 12, 1993, we went to Presbyterian St. Luke's Hospital at 6 AM. We handed Anthony over to Dr.

Victor in the surgical suite, where he began an 11-hour-long surgery. He had a craniotomy and was incised from ear to ear so that his front facial skin could be flipped forward, his upper palate was removed and replaced, and his left cheekbone was displaced and rewired so that as much debulking of the tumor as possible could be done.

The procedure began around 7:30 AM, and Anthony got out of surgical recovery around 10 PM. Those were the most extended 14&1/2 hours of my entire life. Each second of that moment felt like a century.

We paced back and forth, praying and hoping things would work out. But indeed, God sends help in the most unexpected ways.

At the hospital, I met a beautiful Christian woman, Linda, who I believe was an angel sent from above. She was from Nebraska and had come to visit a coworker's son. Linda had a beautiful voice and was a divine intervention for our family. She sang magnificently, played guitar, and prayed with us, which provided a source of consolation. She spent a lot of time with us at the hospital over the next few days.

Linda was also one of the many signs that God was with us on this intense journey of the unknown. Her calm and soothing voice gave me inner peace. Her presence gave us **HOPE** and comfort when we needed it the most.

After the procedure, Anthony was shifted to the Intensive Care Unit. He was on a respirator, and his face was swollen like a bowling ball; stitches were all over his scalp, intravenous lines and drainage tubes were everywhere, and a tracheostomy was in place.

Never did I imagine my story would also have these heartbreaking flashes. When I looked at Anthony, it felt like someone had grasped my heart so hard that I almost could not breathe. Tony and I couldn't watch this happening to our baby boy. We were broken and crying for his recovery. And it was the first time Tony's father had cried.

Tony always mentioned how his father was a strong man, so watching his father shed tears over Anthony's condition was surprising. His dad, Joe, a retired state trooper, was very attached to Anthony and spent a lot of time with him. He even arranged a visit to the fire station where Anthony was on the local news as the little boy with cancer and was lifted high on the firetruck with his grandpa.

We were all seeking a response from Dr. Victor after the surgery. We just wanted to hear those few words that would change our fate forever. Finally, the doctor showed up with mixed expressions. We couldn't tell what he was about to say.

But he said what we **HOPED** for: "Though complicated and long, the surgery was a success!"

We breathed a huge sigh of relief as soon as he completed his sentence. Those words were like a lifeline, not just for our little boy but also for us as a family. I felt so grateful to God at that moment. All our prayers and efforts had finally paid off.

The surgery turned out to be a success with the help of support and prayers from our families. My heart finally began to find solace. This victory belonged not only to Tony and me but to our families as well. They took care of every matter that we had left behind in Erie. Not only that, our parents stood next to us throughout our stay in Denver.

Having lost over 1 liter of blood from the surgery, Anthony was very weak and spent one week in the intensive care unit. And seeing him in this condition was extremely difficult. Yet we kept our **HOPES** up and strengthened our faith in God. We knew He could make things better for us.

I always believed my little Anthony was a superhero like his dad. He constantly kept running back to life regardless of his misfortunes. With God's will, Anthony recovered with resiliency after a few weeks. He got better sooner than the doctors expected. Before Anthony had gone in for the surgery, we happened to meet a rhabdomyosarcoma survivor. He was a young boy who had chosen radiation therapy. Due to that, he was facing some side effects, as we predicted for Anthony.

He told us, "I have to wear a nasal cannula of oxygen at bedtime."

Though his survival through the treatment protocol for RMS was successful, we could not help but think of the complications that radiotherapy would bring.

Tony and I made a courageous and challenging decision by going against what all the leading authorities had recommended. We vowed not to radiate to avoid as many side effects as possible so that if he lived, he would live an everyday healthy life.

At Anthony's young age, we were concerned about multiple complications that could occur, like learning disabilities, cataracts, facial asymmetry and deformity, and stunted growth since the tumor was close to his pituitary gland.

After the surgery, Anthony had to go through sessions of chemotherapy again. We stayed in Denver while he completed his treatment, but it was for an extended period. So, we decided to head back to Erie to continue the maintenance chemotherapy for nine more months.

The maintenance chemotherapy was not as harsh as the first three months of induction chemotherapy. Anthony tolerated the doses better and experienced fewer side effects and infections. But his biggest challenge was becoming a toddler again. Although Anthony was recovering steadily from the surgery, I felt that the children of his age had left him behind. His condition brought on a lot of change in his nature. He was often quiet and only involved in playing with baby Ginelle. Tony and I worried about his behavior, yet knew he had been through a lot that no one his age could bear. But still, we wanted him to recover physically and emotionally. We wanted him to live typically like any other toddler.

We never gave up **HOPE** for a miracle. We had to trust God above all else, even when life's events seemed to sever us from all that would give meaning and **HOPE** to living. We had to trust God enough to let go of our own lives and that of our loved ones.

*"Rejoice in **HOPE**, be patient in tribulation, be constant in prayer."*

(Romans 12:12)

And we did! We trusted God enough to leave Anthony's future in His loving and compassionate arms. Giving it all to God does not mean everything turns out fine. Jesus was quick to reinforce what experience has already taught us: life involves excruciating pain.

Being followers of Jesus does not make us immune to tragedy or difficulty. Nor does it make suffering or death easier, in the physical and emotional sense. Even Jesus prayed, "Let this cup pass." Yet He put himself in God's hands and went through death on a cross for our sake, so we do not have to go alone into the unknown. Jesus beckons us in (**Matthew 16:24-25):**

"If anyone desires to come after Me, let him deny himself, and take up his cross, and follow Me."

Jesus has gone ahead of us, not instead of us. There are no easy answers to the dilemmas and terrors in our lives. Yet, in the midst of it all, the Lord of Life calls us to follow Him and walk with Him. We boast for the **HOPE** and glory in our sufferings because we know that hard times produce perseverance, character, and **HOPE**. It does not put us to shame because God's love has been poured out into our hearts through the Holy Spirit, who has been given to us.

Chapter 5: Rare Recurrence

HOPE Rx *"Not only so, but we also glory in our sufferings because we know that suffering produces perseverance; perseverance, character; and character, **HOPE**."*

(Romans 5:3-4)

As a family, we were exhausted, especially our little boy, Anthony. Unlike a regular toddler, he had been through so much. We were concerned about his life. We didn't want him to feel left out.

Anthony did go into remission in the Spring of 1994 after completion of one year of chemotherapy with the skull-based surgery sandwiched in between. During the year of remission, my family clung to our faith. We knew God would never disappoint us, even in the darkest times. He has His ways of doing things, which we cannot always comprehend. After surviving chemotherapy for almost a year, it was time to take a break from all of it.

Our family had gone through the completion of Tony's residency, the birth of baby Ginelle, and Anthony's recovery, which made our lives busy and purposeful. We needed this time to recuperate, recalibrate, and breathe fresh air.

I was grateful to God for every moment I spent with my family. It was something I had strongly desired for a long time—an escape from all the worries and fears. We had finally received our miracle, or so we thought. We were one year out since Anthony's last round of chemotherapy. It was hard to believe that Anthony's first diagnosis happened two years ago.

I had **HOPE** to see him grow old with his family. But my confidence began to shatter when Anthony appeared with some unexpected symptoms in early March 1995. At four-and-a-half years old, he started to experience breathing complications, shortness of breath and mouth breathing, fatigue, tummy aches, dizziness, loss of appetite, anemia, and coughing. Each symptom built a wave of suspicion within us, so we took Anthony to the hospital for testing.

The results left us stunned.

After many tests and scans in Pittsburgh, a three-by-six-centimeter mass in Anthony's right lung was revealed. We were on the brink of crumbling from such horrible news. That was when the following verse became a reality for us.

"Then the earth shook and trembled; The foundations also of the hills moved and were shaken, because he was wroth. There went up a smoke out of his nostrils, And fire out of his mouth devoured: Coals were kindled by it."

(Psalms 18:7-8)

Where did we go wrong? We thought we had made good decisions concerning Anthony's treatment plan. We decided to head back to Denver to see the pediatric oncologist immediately for a second opinion. But before our expedition, we saw our church family at the 1st Assembly of God in Erie during Sunday services. It was a brand-new pastor's first sermon at our church on that particular Sunday. We tearfully requested our friends to supplicate and said, "We really need your prayers." It was not easy to start these intense treatments all over again. We had just recovered from the trauma. We were so discouraged as we had already put Anthony through so much of an ordeal, and it didn't work as planned. It was time to explore other options.

On March 5, 1995, my family finally reached Denver to get Anthony evaluated. The oncology team suggested an MRI to get a better visualization. While the technicians performed the MRI, I questioned God and His plans. I must admit I felt as though God had betrayed me because this was not what we had prayed and **HOPED** for.

It was heartbreaking for me as a mother to let my son go through the torture again and again. My heart couldn't stop questioning God about all this. After the surgery, I thought it was the end of suffering for my son, but I was wrong. I was disappointed in God as I couldn't understand His strategies.

But then I pulled myself up and prayed to God for Anthony's ease and comfort. It was an Abraham and Isaac experience, but our altar was the MRI table. I had to trust and relinquish Anthony again to God's Almighty hands.

The results of the MRI were not promising. Anthony's prognosis was poorer than before, and he had a less than 5% chance of long-term survival. The oncology team gave no **HOPE** and instead instructed us to palliate Anthony with narcotics until he passed.

I couldn't help but think: *Is this for real?* After all the effort to keep him alive, all they wanted was to let him go. He was my son, Anthony, they were talking about! How could we possibly let this happen? He had been through hell and lost his innocence, all for a chance to live.

We would not accept the palliation idea. *As long as there is breath, there is **HOPE**.* Furthermore, human calculations have no place with God.

Tony and I were adamant and refused to proceed with that suggestion. We were determined to at least attempt further treatments to check if Anthony would respond positively.

The oncology team gave us the most distressing news—more than anything we could have dreamed. Anthony's cancer, Rhabdomyosarcoma, was now at Stage 4, having metastasized into his right lung. That report completely shattered my dreams when I was finally comfortable with the idea that a perfect life with my family was possible.

The doctors suggested several biopsies to rule out the nature of the tumor. In addition, they performed a five-hour surgery that included a thoracoscopic lung biopsy and two bone marrow biopsies. At the end of the procedure, they placed a chest tube in Anthony.

Not only this, but our son also went through several minor surgeries, which included inserting a double-lumen Broviac catheter into the vein through his skin so that Anthony could receive more chemotherapy in Pittsburgh.

While we were in Denver, Dr. Victor biopsied and cleaned out Anthony's sinuses. If there was any silver lining to this whole experience, it was that the tumor had not spread to other parts of his body, according to the numerous tests and scans performed. These minor tests and surgeries made Anthony fragile, so we stayed in Denver until his recovery. But once he was stable, we moved back to Pittsburgh to figure out the next step in his treatment.

The doctors in Pittsburgh suggested harsher and more aggressive chemotherapy drugs to eradicate the tumor. They also recommended having a lung wedge resection of the tumor and a stem cell transplant to maximize Anthony's chance of survival.

Oh gosh! Do we really want to put him through all this torture again? This idea kept nagging us while we were on the verge of making the right decision. We were perplexed; regardless of all the medical knowledge, choosing the best option for our son was agonizing.

We sought help and counseling from our pastor as we needed a perspective of faith. He guided us, stating, "It would be appropriate to start the chemotherapy and see if Anthony responded positively. If he did, that would be a sign to continue the treatments that we were dreading." He was a great support, which we desperately needed at that moment.

When we were in Denver, our oncology team had warned us that the disease progression was far worse than the treatment. Therefore, we were vigilant with every minute detail. We wanted to defeat it for Anthony, but we were heartbroken because he had to start another year of chemotherapy.

In March 1995, after Easter, amid all the stress and anxiety, I discovered that I was expecting our third child. This was exciting news for our family—it gave us **HOPE** and optimism. Tony and I wanted to share the news with our firstborn, Anthony, before informing anyone else. Anthony got so happy, and, in all the exhilaration, he gave me a big hug that made my heart cry.

He prayed to God, "Jesus, take all the bad things away, and don't let the new baby get sick." Anthony's toddler years were anything but average, but his resilience, tolerance, and stamina were unbelievable. His faith in God alone was astonishing; he often used to say, "Jesus is stronger than Superman. Heaven is beautiful. Jesus loves me more than anyone else. Mommy, what will you do if Jesus gives you another boy and takes me away to heaven?"

I had no answer to his questions. I knew nothing about the future. All I had was **HOPE** for a better ending— especially for Anthony's sake. We were exhausted by every standard option and wanted a suitable one for our son. It was time to go to the world's end to look for natural alternative cancer treatments.

I called every pediatric transplant center in the country, consulting with countless pediatric oncologists on whether an autologous or allogeneic transplant would be best for our son.

The allogeneic transplant had more risks of graft-versus-host disease, whereas the autologous transplant (from Anthony's own body) risked reinfusing cancerous cells back into his body. We chose to go with the autologous transplant.

We needed prayers like never before to make this work at any cost. Submitting our worries to God made everything so much easier.

"He performs wonders that cannot be fathomed, miracles that cannot be counted." **(Job 5:9)**

Once again, the Lord reminded me of the rhema word that I clung to in **(Psalm 118:17): "***I shall not die, but live, and declare the works of the Lord.***"**

Chapter 6: The Transplant

HOPE Rx *"And **HOPE** does not put us to shame, because God's love has been poured out into our hearts through the Holy Spirit, who has been given to us."*

(Romans 5:5)

There is tremendous power in **HOPE** and faith, and this was the fuel that drove us to persevere once again. This feeling of assurance is undoubtedly a sign from God that He hasn't given up on us, and so we shouldn't give up either.

With all the dependence on the mercy of God, we started the cycle of heavy-duty chemotherapy once again. The potential side effects included infections, hemorrhaging, organ failure, and possible death.

Anthony spent most of his time at the hospital so the doctor could monitor every detail. The four-week cycle of induction chemotherapy was critical. The doctors kept preparing us for the worst as if a less than 5% chance of survival was not enough to discourage us. The high doses of cancer treatment before a stem cell transplant can cause several problems, such as bleeding, increased risk of infection, mouth sores, nausea, fevers, and extreme fatigue. And so, it happened with these repercussions.

On June 6, 1995, Anthony underwent a four-hour wedge resection of his right lung with two chest tubes placed. At last, there was some light in the darkness, and our oncologist, Dr. Michael, gave us good news, reporting: "The preliminary pathology showed that none of the biopsies taken had a viable tumor." We decided not to go for radiation once again and proceed with the stem cell transplant. We got through the 1st four significant rounds of chemotherapy and started preparing for the stem cell transplant.

There are essentially three steps to an autologous stem cell transplant. First, blood is withdrawn from the patient and passed through a machine that separates the stem cells, which are then frozen and stored. This is called the harvesting. The second step is the patient receives very high doses of chemotherapy to kill the cancer cells and prepare the body for the transplant. This process is called conditioning and can last one to seven days. The last step is transplanting, which is when the stem cells are thawed and infused back into the patient intravenously. The stem cells then migrate to the bone marrow and begin producing normal blood cells after about two weeks. After the transplant, the patient must stay in the hospital for at least one month until the blood counts are safe and must return for regular checkups.

Our lives just became more intense and complicated. After thorough research and discussions, we finalized the date for our son's transplant as it was the best option with the best chances. This verse helped us out in those dark times:

"And those who mourn are lifted to safety."

(Job 5:11)

On June 21, 1995, Anthony was admitted to Children's Hospital in Pittsburgh for a stem cell transplant. A device similar to a dialysis machine was used to remove blood cells from Anthony's body. Then Anthony received very high doses of chemotherapy, which were approximately 4 ½ times the normal doses and nearly lethal.

My son's life became a continuous ride from the hospital to home and back. *Why couldn't our little guy just enjoy an innocent childhood? Why did he have to be robbed of his innocence at such a young age?*

The autologous bone marrow transplant was performed on June 30, 1995. Tony and I didn't let go of each other and prayed constantly. We were optimistic about the autologous transplant because it involved cells from Anthony's body and carried less risk of complications. Things didn't go as smoothly as we anticipated.

Several complications hit Anthony hard. In the oncology unit, he acquired a nosocomial rotavirus infection, which led to severe nausea, vomiting, and diarrhea for a total of six months.

He was supposed to receive a platelet transfusion as his platelet count was very low, but the doctor decided against it. Consequently, our son began hemorrhaging from the rectum, causing him to lose over 1 liter of blood a day for eight consecutive days. He went into hemorrhagic shock and spent 2 1/2 weeks on a respirator in the ICU with no white cell count. Both of his lungs collapsed, and he developed Veno-Occlusive Disease (VOD) of the liver.

According to the literature, only fifty percent of people recover from VOD, and the other fifty percent develop encephalopathy and die.

During this time in the ICU, Anthony received countless blood and platelet transfusions and fluids to keep him alive. The doctors induced a coma with medication for three weeks to keep him comfortable. The storms of complications raged against our family's efforts to save our son. By then, Anthony required a nasogastric NG tube for bowel drainage.

Seeing our son in that condition, hooked up to tubes, surrounded by beeping machines and medical staff, was overwhelming. Not only that, but I was pregnant with our third child and had to watch this play out hour by hour in the ICU.

I appealed desperately for prayers from all our relatives, friends, and church family. The Sunday evening services were in progress at Erie First Assembly, where a couple of hundred people were in attendance that night. They rose from their pews and joined hands, forming a circle inside the church, to audibly cry out together in prayer for Anthony.

By God's grace, the prayers worked! My son began to graft cells into his own body after eight days and miraculously made it out of the ICU even though the medical staff presumed that he would not. Though I was happy to see his progress, it was devastating to watch our little boy lose all his muscle tone and not have enough strength to talk for 2 1/2 weeks.

The doctors thought he was suffering from a narcotic overdose, so they administered anti-narcotic agents to attempt to reverse the mutism. *Or could this mutism possibly be from ICU psychosis?* It was hard to tell. Occupational therapists worked with Anthony, and soon, he began talking again and regained some of his strength.

"Thank you, Jesus!!!!" was all I could think, say, and pray.

The doctors predicted that Anthony would have to stay in the hospital for up to 100 days after the transplant, but he was discharged after two months. I remember when Anthony stepped into his bedroom again; he was so happy and thankful for this blessing. He prayed, "Thank you, Jesus, for bringing me home from the hospital."

I have never seen a boy so little yet mature enough to understand everything happening around him. Although Anthony was home, his intravenous and tube feedings continued for six months. I was a full-time nurse, a part-time mother to Ginelle, and a very part-time wife to Tony.

As I said before, our families were a great help during this time of need. And once again, my brother came to our rescue. One day, he showed up at the Children's Hospital with a brand-new blue minivan so we could run Anthony's IVs and tube feedings on our trips back and forth from Pittsburgh. Our new van served the purpose of a mini hospital, but I couldn't have been more thankful for it.

Anthony was still fighting with post-transplant complications. He hadn't recovered from the virus he had encountered back at the hospital. We even tried IV gamma globulin for six weeks to cure the rotavirus, but no positive outcome resulted.

Eventually, things started to look up. I will never forget my birthday on September 9, 1995. It was my 35th birthday, and I got an amazing phone call from the lab indicating Anthony's complete clearance of the virus. It was the best birthday present ever. My little boy was finally relieved!

The virus cure came from donated breast milk we introduced into the feeding tube. I was still pregnant, so I did not yet produce breast milk. Two generous women from our church family came forward to help, as did my sister-in-law.

While celebrating the clearance of the virus for my son, I realized that my due date was near—it was December 24, 1995. To avoid any inconvenience, we deliberately planned an early follow-up visit to Anthony's doctor in Pittsburgh for peace of mind before the birth of our third child.

On December 1, we headed to Pittsburgh. I remember I became very weak and nauseous that day. I overlooked all the signs and considered it a viral flu as I was focused on my son's checkup. The hospital staff even commented that I did not look well. After the checkup, we returned to Erie. On our way back, my symptoms aggravated. *Could I possibly be in labor 21 days early?* That night, I got admitted to the hospital for what we thought was just false labor or a bad flu.

The staff administered intravenous fluids to stop the contractions, but that did not work.

It turned out I was in full-blown labor again. We were worried about Anthony, so we asked his grandpa to come over and look after him. Tony and I wanted Anthony to witness the birth of another sibling. So, our little guy disconnected his tube all by himself and came to the delivery room with Tony's father.

This time, I suffered more than usual because I had the flu on top of my labor. Anthony witnessed every moment of giving birth to his younger brother.

After much hassle and pain, I gave birth to my third child, Anthony's baby brother, Victor Anthony. The name Victor Anthony signified "*Victory for Anthony.*" I chose this name because it's always been special to me. My brother, who died in the tragic accident, and the surgeon who performed Anthony's surgery in Denver shared the same name. They were very important men to me, and I wanted my son Victor to be their namesake. The name Victor means "*Conqueror,*" and Anthony means "*Priceless.*"

As Anthony stayed in the delivery room, he was disturbed by the pain I was going through to bring a child into the world.

He told his daddy, "I don't want Mommy to have any more babies."

His reaction confused Tony, who asked, "Why is that?"

Anthony replied, "Because that was way too hard for mommy."

I had just seen Anthony, our little boy, battle for every breath of his life for three solid weeks. Not only that, he had been battling for his life throughout most of his early years, yet there he was, empathizing with my pain. He was so gentle during the birthing, gently rubbing my hand and encouraging me beautifully. How could I say that this natural childbirth was hard for me, knowing everything my son had just been through? After what our little trooper experienced, how dare I complain?

After the transplant, Anthony was still susceptible to infections because his immune system was not strong enough to fight all the pathogens. This required Anthony to keep a distance from children who recently received live vaccines like chicken pox or oral polio, so he could not attend regular preschool. We started privately tutoring him for preschool, which began a whole new chapter for our boy.

After adding baby Victor to our family, we sensed a new direction in our lives. We began to move forward in our reality—Anthony had a sister and a brother to grow up with now.

In the Fall of 1996, Anthony entered Kindergarten with 23 other boys and girls. They became his close friends and made him feel like a normal child.

*"But those who **HOPE** in the Lord will renew their strength. They will soar on wings like eagles; they will run and not grow weary. They will walk and not be faint."*

(Isaiah 40:31)

Chapter 7: Powerful Prayers

HOPE Rx *"Let us hold unswervingly to the **HOPE** we profess, for He who promised is faithful."*

(Hebrews 10:23)

The trajectory of my life was often an unanticipated path. Sometimes, it was like I was part of a marathon I did not sign up for. Sometimes, it was like I was in a never-ending race, constantly running to figure out a way to make it home safely.

Though it seemed like a dream, God always helped me on my journey. He repeatedly showed His signs along the way, feeding my **HOPE**. It didn't matter if I felt lost on the track. He would perk up the skies for me whenever there was no light.

My family had faced numerous challenges and endured an incredible amount of pain. On a Sunday morning in June 1996, when our son Victor was six months old and being dedicated at our church, a rather unexpected event occurred.

We were planning a big family gathering to celebrate Victor's baby dedication, and our close friend, Linda from Nebraska, flew in to be his godmother. My family was driving up from West Virginia for this celebration. But as I was bathing Victor, I noticed little petechiae and bruises all over his skin and inside his mouth. I called my friend, a doctor, and she advised me to take him to the emergency room immediately. I was going to see the doctor on Monday and wondered if this could wait. But she said no.

The dedication didn't occur at our church; instead, it happened in the emergency room of our local hospital with our senior pastor. We had to carefully drive to Pittsburgh Children's Hospital to have Victor admitted since it was too difficult to start intravenous meds in Erie due to his extremely low platelet count of 2000. It was discovered that Victor had Idiopathic Thrombocytopenic Purpura (ITP). This rare condition occurs when the spleen does not recognize the platelets, viewing them as foreign bodies and eating them up.

We had to carefully wrap Victor's head to protect him from any bumps on the two-hour drive to Children's Hospital. The doctor was concerned Victor had leukemia, and I thought: *What is the likelihood of having two sons with cancer?*

When the nurses saw the name "Victor Anthony Ruffa" at the oncology unit, they assumed it was Anthony again. Victor had to receive platelet transfusions and gamma globulin to raise his platelet count over several days. Thankfully, it was not leukemia, and we never had to remove his spleen.

After the completion of Anthony's stem cell transplant, he was required to have repeated follow-ups in Pittsburgh every three months. Each time, it was a complete set of tests, including CT scans and MRI of the head and neck. This was fatiguing for our son as he needed a break from all of this.

We wanted a moment to ourselves, too—at least to pretend we were a normal family. We wanted to forget what had happened to our baby Anthony. We wanted to appreciate this time and be grateful to God that our precious boy was still alive and with us. My family decided to take a vacation to Disney World in February 1998 over the winter break to relax and drain away all the negative thoughts ever present in our minds.

Shortly after our vacation in February 1998, when Anthony was in first grade at Erie First Assembly of God school, he began showing symptoms, including a lingering cough and shortness of breath, which concerned us. We consulted his pediatrician hastily, as we didn't want to waste a minute. He was worried and referred us to Children's Hospital in Pittsburgh for further testing. It was as concerning for us as it was for the doctor.

The ENT doctor in Erie placed Anthony on antibiotics to see if his symptoms would improve. A telephone prayer chain was started among our family members and friends at the church. We were in dire need of prayers from everyone. We were not prepared to hear anything disturbing again. This episode of symptoms was five years from the date of Anthony's original diagnosis. I didn't tremble and sought courage from God as I knew only He could handle this matter. Church friends did an intercessory prayer for us by doing Jericho marches for Anthony when things were very critical. In March 1998, the boys and girls from Anthony's class joined the fight for his life.

I could sense what our son was going through; I wanted to resolve all his difficulties. But it was only conceivable by trusting in God and His plans. Once, while we were heading toward Pittsburgh for Anthony's follow-up, he kept staring at the sky.

Curious, I couldn't resist asking him, "What are you looking at?"

Anthony didn't look at me because he was perplexed and consumed by his thoughts; instead, he maintained eye contact with the sky as if he were watching something happen up there.

I tried again, "Anthony, what are you looking at?"

He replied, "*I can see the gates of heaven opening up, and the gates open when someone dies.*"

Anthony's words pierced my heart. My impression of the gates of heaven opening up was that it welcomed Anthony's soul from his earthly life to a heavenly home and that heaven must be preparing for his arrival. I was speechless when he uttered those words. He was just a little boy who had suffered so much torment. I couldn't imagine how he had been psychologically dealing with all those fears.

He could see through things beyond imagination. We had repeatedly traveled the road from Erie to Pittsburgh, yet that trip seemed the longest. It's a part of the country where overcast skies are common, but that day, it wasn't the cloudy skies that dampened my spirits.

"Be strong and courageous… for the Lord your God goes with you. The Lord Himself goes before you and will be with you; He will never leave you nor forsake you. Do not be afraid; do not be discouraged."

(Deuteronomy 31:6-8)

We went to Pittsburgh for further diagnosis, which turned out to be unfavorable for us. The results showed another mass in Anthony's right lung, 2 x 3 cm in size. That news shattered every expectation I had and even made Anthony cry. He asked if it was cancer.

He questioned, *"Why did Jesus let my cancer come back after we prayed so hard to get rid of it?"* He wanted to know why he always had to get needles in his arms and cancer.

We initially received the news of Anthony's cancer on March 13, 1993, and his lung recurrence in March 1995. If it were not for this lung mass diagnosis on March 13, 1998, Anthony would have been considered at the 5-year mark of being cancer-free. But fate's plans are different from what we desire. This update on Anthony's health knocked us way off balance and almost took away our will to move on. It was the hopelessness that had rung in the voice of the oncologist who had just delivered to us the prognosis for Anthony's third bout with cancer: untreatable.

Hearing that news for the third time was intense enough to crush our hearts. Tony and I were lost; it was such a crushing blow to us as parents because when it's your child, everything changes. We felt helplessness and despair; we both were disheartened about that diagnosis.

Haven't we had enough shock and disbelief? How many more tear-filled sleepless nights? It seemed impossible. Just a few months before, we experienced a renewal of our faith. We had always gone to church, but we had become more aware of God's personal interest in our lives and more impressed with a desire to commit all areas of our lives to honoring and serving Him. We anticipated the abundant life that the Scriptures promise. Instead, we began our way through that "dark tunnel," searching for a way to break cancer's grip on our curly-headed toddler. I journaled during this time, expressing how bitter, overwhelmed, discouraged, frustrated, and miserable I was. I wondered how God could ever put us back together again with all these broken pieces. This news felt dehumanizing, humbling, and humiliating. Our reserves were so low this third time around.

The doctors were not giving us **HOPE** this time. According to them: "The disease is very aggressive and rampant; he is going to die."

Instead of boosting our confidence, they constantly said this to us for two and a half weeks.

The treatment options that were suggested were not promising enough and were only offering temporary control or some degree of comfort from the excruciating pain that was to be expected as the disease advanced.

I could see Anthony losing his confidence with each passing second. He lamented to both of us, *"It's just not fair. Why do I have to get cancer?"*

Those questions were not blamable; only Jesus could respond to them by blessing us with a surprise. This situation was entirely out of our hands now. All my years of knowledge and research work were gone in vain. We could not decide what else to do at this point.

(Psalm 73:26)" *My flesh and my heart may fail, but God is the strength of my heart and my portion forever."*

Anthony's teachers began to collect resources to help his classmates cope with the predicted loss of their friend when the time came. One of the friends stood before their congregation and requested prayer for Anthony's long and healthy life.

At the Erie First Assembly, our pastor was kind and understood our situation very well. He led the adults and youth in prayer for Anthony in the main sanctuary the Sunday morning after the diagnosis. The children's director played melodies of faith on her guitar. In contrast, almost 100 children knelt at the altar in the chapel and prayed for Anthony's healing during the children's service.

I could compare my feelings to the time when I first became aware of the cancer. It was actually more difficult the third time because we had already gone through this not only once but twice, and three times was just too much to tolerate. I felt betrayed by God and wondered: *Why couldn't Anthony's previous recovery be the end of our trial?*

My sentiments were not the way they used to be; I went into severe depression for almost three weeks. I had a fear that not only could cancer come back, but it did come back, and this time with a vengeance. Anthony used to ask me, "Are you going to cry, Mommy, when I die?" Or, he would say something like, "Mommy, will you always be with me forever, whenever I go to heaven? I want Mommy, Daddy, and Belly (Ginelle) to be with me in heaven."

I was a miserable wreck. I gathered all the possible information regarding Anthony's treatment, yet I was still on the same page where it all began. I was disappointed, but then I realized that I could not be mad at God for letting this happen. I would have to accept and trust Him, regardless of the circumstances and outcome. I had to believe in God's plan despite how discouraged I was. There was no time to pity ourselves. We just had to do what we could to get through this.

I asked myself: *Who am I to question God's plan and purpose?* His plans are always better than mine. His love for Anthony is far greater than mine, for sure. I needed to submit to Him in faith. I could not comprehend it, and even if I could, I was unwilling to accept what he had in store for us. I had to go through that valley at any cost. Pastor knew the depth of our situation. He assisted me in those hard times and showed me a way out by giving references from the Bible:

"Yea, though I walk through the valley of the shadow of death, I will fear no evil: for thou art with me; Thy rod and thy staff, they comfort me."

(Psalm 23:4)

He elaborated on this verse for me to encourage my faith. In his opinion, there was an entrance and an exit to this valley experience, and all of it was temporary. I recognized that I could not just stand at one point; I had to go *through* the valley.

It seemed as though my whole world revolved around the word *CANCER*. That's all I could relate to, and it consumed our lives. I had a tough time listening to the lives, routines, and measly complaints of normal families. Because when I used to compare mine with theirs, a valid discrepancy was evident.

With a heavy heart and soul, my family packed and traveled to Pittsburgh yet again for the surgical removal of the tumor.

On arrival, I requested the doctors to perform a CT scan of my son's chest one more time before moving on with the surgery. I had a gut feeling there was a chance of some good news as we noticed a few improvements in Anthony's symptoms following a course of antibiotics.

*"Be strong and take heart, all you who **HOPE** in the Lord."*

(Psalm 31:24)

After a lot of persuasion, the hospital staff reluctantly granted my request. They performed a CT scan and canceled the surgery. I wondered if they made this decision because the cancer metastasized in the body and was now considered inoperable. Surprisingly, the results elated us.

The CT scan showed no tumor or mass! What had been there could have been pneumonia, which had resolved with antibiotics. Or, we received another miracle from God.

The doctors sent us home and just advised us to follow up on the suspicious nodule. The news was a great relief. We were eager to share it with my family, so we traveled to West Virginia to celebrate the event with a pizza party and Nintendo games before returning to Erie. I told Anthony we better thank Jesus, and he said, *"I already did."*

I told him it was the best news ever, and he responded by saying, "The best news ever was when I really did have cancer, and Jesus took it away."

We returned home and decided to share our journey with friends and family at the church. I spent the next day on the phone relaying our great news to everyone.

On Sunday, Tony and I stood up before our congregation. I was holding up a briefcase packed with five years of research on Anthony's condition and told everyone, "I feel like God is telling me that I don't need this anymore."

But I still wondered: *What about the gates of heaven that Anthony saw on the way home from Pittsburgh after this third-time cancer revelation?*

A good friend of mine and prayer partner, Tracy, prayed intensely after hearing our family was going through a third cancer scare with Anthony.

While praying, she read these verses where an angel tells Daniel:

"Your words were heard, and I have come in response to them."

(Daniel 10:12-13)

My friend saw angels leaving the gates of heaven to do battle on Anthony's behalf. This explanation for Anthony's steady stare at the sky made sense. I got my answers; they were the angels who moved out from the gates to help and save the life of my precious little boy.

"But as for you ye thought evil against me; but God meant it unto good, to bring to pass, as it is this day, to save many people alive."

(Genesis 50:20)

"Bless the Lord, O my soul, and forget not all His benefits: Who forgives all your iniquities, who heals all your diseases, who redeems your life from destruction, who crowns you with lovingkindness and tender mercies, who satisfies your mouth with good things, so that your youth is renewed like the eagle's."

(Psalm 103:2-5)

Chapter 8: Holistic Healing

HOPE Rx *"Now the God of **HOPE** fill you with all joy and peace in believing, that ye may abound in **HOPE,** through the power of the Holy Ghost."*

(Romans 15:13)

With each moment passing, my faith in God became stronger. I never imagined I could handle this all on my own, but with God's amazing grace, I did. I was keeping everything together for my family out of sheer necessity. I sensed a different energy in my body; it was so influential that it really kept me going. I was on an unstoppable mission.

I believe God only gives us the amount of suffering we can tolerate and no more. He wouldn't let us go through any turmoil without making us able to learn something out of it. He wouldn't permit us to grieve without sharing with others what we have learned through our trials and tribulations. The comfort that comes from God through these challenging trials is undeniable.

There are mainly two ways to seek liberation from all sicknesses; the first is intercessory prayer, and the second is medical intervention. I believe these two modalities and consistent prayer helped Anthony the most in his recovery journey from cancer. I believe the two most valuable holistic interventions for Anthony were juicing and breast milk.

Being a pharmacist, I was aware of all the medicines and their potential adverse effects on health. The medicines can drastically affect the physical and emotional health of a child.

Therefore, I was hypervigilant with Anthony's diet. I had to monitor and look thoroughly at his diet plan. After years of research and hard work, I realized that food was the medicine to reverse Anthony's condition. I learned that food had all the key components to make his life better and healthy. I started this nutritional journey not only for Anthony but for my other kids as well.

Fruits and vegetables have all the necessary phytochemicals to help the body avoid harmful foreign substances and also help boost the immune system. Hence, I began making fresh fruit and vegetable juices every morning and evening, regularly and religiously, and fed them to Anthony and my other children. In fact, the kids were not allowed to play with friends or go to after-school events until they drank their juice. Mama G was the "Juice Nazi."

I had to beg and plead with the doctors to insert a feeding tube into Anthony, and they very reluctantly granted my request. This made the challenging situation less problematic. We started out with a nasogastric (NG) tube, but I later had the doctors change it to a nasojejunal (NJ) tube to bypass the stomach and get to the small intestine. This allowed for better absorption of the nutrients. I drew all the juices into a syringe and attached it to the feeding tube with a luer lock to get the nutrients into his body. It was very satisfying for me because I could see all the liquid nourishment entering his body, and it helped me witness the transitions in his health. I also read several articles on the benefits of breast milk in curing several diseases and increasing the body's self-defense. Breast milk has many powerful compounds, including lactoferrin, which is an antibacterial and antiviral protein that is instrumental in establishing the infant's immune system. Milk fat globule membrane (MFGM) is a combination of lipids and proteins in breast milk, which is nutrient-rich and provides important immune, respiratory, and cognitive development support for newborns during the first weeks of life. Colostrum also contains anticarcinogenic properties that kill tumor-producing cells and immunoglobulins that assist in rebuilding the gut, which is our second immune system. Before Victor's birth, I decided to feed Anthony breast milk, too. I gave it to Anthony through the feeding tube to fortify his immune system. It was Tony's job to retrieve the donated milk from our donors. We often joked about the situation and chuckled, saying, "The milkman is here."

After Victor's birth, we no longer had to request milk from donors, as I was able to share the breast milk between Anthony and Victor. But I am forever grateful for the generosity and kindness of our donors. The breast milk helped cure Anthony's six months of rotavirus, which he had acquired in the hospital. Investigating all the alternatives for cancer treatment was entirely exhausting and overwhelming because the options were endless. Being a mother and a pharmacist, I had to figure out the best treatment that would resonate with my mind and heart, which clearly was a lot of pressure. God said:

"I give you every seed-bearing plant on the face of the whole earth and every tree that has fruit with seed in it. They will be yours for food."

(Genesis 1:29)

I read every article imaginable stating the merits of shark cartilage, miracles of mistletoe, and odd things like hydrazine sulfate injections and everything else from A to Z, including apricot kernels, castor oil packs, and coffee enemas. I learned a lot along the way but had to weigh the benefits vs. the risks and sift through endless information with caution and **HOPE**.

The juicing method was a no-brainer; it was a simple and efficient method to get five to nine servings of fresh vegetables in a juice to be provided to the body of our four-year-old son in a very assimilable fashion. We would have to chew a serving of fruits, vegetables, or salad at least 50 times to get the same amount of nutrients that you get from drinking a sip of freshly squeezed juice.

"Let thy food be thy medicine, and thy medicine be thy food."

(Hippocrates)

There is no comparison between the wonders of natural substances and pharmaceuticals. The mechanism of action differs for both treatment approaches. Each fruit and vegetable has unique phytochemicals that support the killing of cancer cells through various processes.

After the stem cell transplant, Anthony lost so much weight and needed good nourishment. He was only four years old when the doctor inserted the feeding tube. I really believe the feeding tube helped to save his life and speed up his recovery. The nutrients circumvented his taste buds and got absorbed into his small intestine. The feeding tube made it possible for me to strengthen Anthony with very healthy options in liquid form. Sometimes, it is necessary to advocate for the patient, especially if their food intake is very poor. The feeding tube was instrumental in making Anthony stronger after all the transplant complications. It greatly reduced the number of blood and platelet transfusions he was receiving after the transplant. I used to make green juices regularly without any disruption in the routine. All my children were forced to drink fresh juices while they were under our roof. My other assigned nickname was *Mother Nature*. Trying to feed Anthony without the feeding tube would have been nearly impossible with the rotavirus and chemotherapy-induced nausea.

As Anthony grew up, green smoothies became a great way to incorporate all sorts of superfoods, fruits, and vegetables into a drinkable fashion. Occasionally, I would let Anthony eat like other kids when he used to hang out with his friends. Later, I would make up for it with the healthy juice concoctions using my best friend, the juicer. While modifying our diet, I learned about many other institutions, resources, and organizations for cancer treatments. A few of them included the Gerson Clinic,

Hallelujah Acres, and the Ann Wigmore Institute. As far as I was concerned, when it came to CANCER, the plant kingdom was the ANSWER. I was surprised to see that there really was not anything from the animal kingdom that could help Anthony the way that plants could. So, I shifted my mind toward adopting a whole food plant-based diet (WFPBD) and an organic lifestyle.

I used to tell my kids, "If it's organic, you don't have to panic." I made lots of big, healthy organic salads with many varieties of colors and textures. I believed that if Anthony was GREEN inside, he would be CLEAN inside. This way, we could rebuild the unhealthy cells and maintain the equilibrium in the body by keeping the integrity of the healthy cells. This became my way of doing ongoing plant-based chemotherapy for my peace of mind, helping to keep Anthony's cancer in remission.

Tony and I never wanted to let go of any moment of happiness without a celebration. We knew the value of these tiny moments and their broad impact on memory lane. Every year that passed, we would celebrate Anthony's birthday as a huge celebration of life. It was indeed a time to forget about the unfortunate tragedies that happened to him as a little boy. We didn't want to take his precious life for granted. We were grateful to God for keeping him with us in a healthy and happy state. While reading about new treatment options, I discovered *Pau D'arco tea* as an option. This tea has anti-inflammatory, antioxidant, and immunomodulating properties.

A German biochemist developed the *Budwig diet* in the 1950s, which included eating flaxseed oil mixed with cottage cheese and Concord grape juice. This combination was thought to make omega-3 fatty acids more available to the body's cells. Essiac Tea is Rene Caisse's last name spelled backward. She was the Canadian nurse who formulated a blend of herbs to help cancer, immunity, and detoxification. This tea has gained widespread popularity among natural health enthusiasts. I also incorporated things like Aloe Vera gel into Anthony's smoothies because it is rich in polysaccharides and contains over 75 active compounds to help disrupt tumor growth and keep the immune system strong. It was prudent to take an integrative approach of combining Western treatment possibilities with alternative ones because the latter helped lessen the side effects caused by the former. However, you should not completely overlook the power of praying as it adds the most significant worth to the treatment. The supremacy of **HOPE** is never an understatement. I worked through all of this by clinging to the plan God had for Anthony; surely, He is omniscient and knows what's best for all of us. He was able to cure my son from this terrible disease, and I had a **HOPE** that He would.

"There is no disease incurable to Jesus. He is the Great Physician."

Chapter 9: Bountiful Blessings

HOPE Rx *"But if we **HOPE** for what we do not yet have, we wait for it patiently."*

(Romans 8:25)

Life was passing by quite calmly until one day, on October 27, 1998. I was home doing all the chores, and suddenly, I felt a little unusual. At that moment, I realized that I was bleeding. I got concerned about a miscarriage and asked Tony to take a day off. I was emotionally unstable, and my body was trembling as I assumed a miscarriage. Anxiety settled in the pit of my heart, making me anxious and sending me into a frenzy of sorts. I needed nothing more than a person by my side to console me.

Tony dropped me off at the OB/GYN office and ran home to get the kids on the school bus that morning. After dropping the kids off, he returned to the doctor's office to join me.

I had already been rushed into an ambulance and admitted to the local hospital due to profuse hemorrhaging. It was an unexpected turn of events; my whole body was in a state of shock and shivering because of the sudden, unforeseen loss of blood. I had an emergency dilation, curettage, and evacuation (D&C&E).

Earlier, I had no idea that this would change into a serious situation and that I would have to get blood transfusions.

This lamentable incident happened before the birth of my fourth child; I was 16 weeks pregnant, and this was now my third miscarriage.

When you are about to become a mother, you go through a series of changes, not just physically but psychologically as well. Miscarriages are not easy to deal with; the pain a woman goes through cannot be described in words. One after another, my life was just becoming an enduring challenge. That loss was something I didn't imagine, especially after the transformation I brought into my life by following a healthy diet regime and trying to be as cautious as possible about everything. Even at that crucial time, I didn't lose **HOPE** in the kindness of God; I didn't question His decision and just admitted what fate had there for me.

In May 2000, Anthony was a ten-year-old boy when our family was blessed with another daughter, Giana Gabrielle (Gigi). Giana means, *"God is gracious,"* and Gabrielle means, *"God gives me strength."* I must say Giana brought so much joy and positive energy into our family after the miscarriages, loss, and emptiness.

Her birth on May 12 was my best Mother's Day gift ever. She became a source of bliss and a **HOPE** to our family. It was such a good memory of Anthony and Ginelle as they witnessed her being born, and also for my mother, who was present for Giana's birth with a nurse midwife at the hospital. Ginelle was so thrilled to bring Giana's baby footprints to school for her show and tell that morning.

God always offers the best to His people, as He did in my life. I was depressed after the last miscarriage, but deep down, I knew God had a better plan for me. I knew He would shower me and my family with the most amazing rewards. Then, He blessed me with a beautiful baby girl who gave me another reason to live. Giana's birth was a reflection of God's promise where He said:

"I will repay you for the years the locusts have eaten–the great locust and the young locust, the other locusts and the locust swarm–my great army that I sent among you. You will have plenty to eat until you are full, and you will praise the name of the Lord your God, who has worked wonders for you; never again will my people be shamed. Then you will know that I am in Israel, that I am the Lord your God, and that there is no other; never again will my people be shamed."

(Joel 2:25-27)

Four months after Giana's birth, Tony went to Arizona to attend a medical conference. He planned to celebrate our anniversary there with baby Giana and me. So, I flew separately with Giana to meet up with him. We were looking forward to having some quality family time that week.

But after we arrived, Giana developed a high-grade fever. She was inconsolable and fussy, which was not her usual demeanor. She also started developing photophobia (sensitivity to light).

Tony and I got worried and took her to the emergency room. The doctors told us not to worry as this was a viral illness and advised us to treat her symptoms with Ibuprofen and Tylenol.

No matter what they said, I still had a feeling of doubt. As I was skeptical about her condition, I convinced Tony to consult a pediatrician to clear my mind.

The next day, we took her to the pediatrician, who examined and found fluid in her soft spot (*fontanelle*). She suspected that Giana could either be having meningitis or a cerebral hemorrhage. I was not prepared for something like this. I already had Anthony go through so much and finally get better that I was not ready to face another life-threatening illness with another baby—not with Giana. Feeling helpless, I kept praying profusely to Jesus to help us in these difficult times.

Upon that diagnosis, we had to call an ambulance to take her from the doctor's office to a children's hospital in Arizona. We spent the entire week at the hospital doing a thorough workup, which included culture and sensitivity testing.

This was all God's plan; I am glad that He gave me that instinct to get her checked again. He guided me when I was lost and shattered.

At the hospital, Giana was treated with intravenous antibiotics in case she had bacterial meningitis. It turned out that she had viral meningitis. It was a frightening experience on that trip because this caught us off guard after what we had experienced with Anthony. Giana took around ten days to show improvement in her condition, and then she was healthy enough to fly home with us.

Once more, God proved His faithfulness to our family. As he stated in the Bible, **HOPE** is the confident expectation of what God has promised, and its strength is in His faithfulness.

"When you go through deep waters and great trouble, I will be with you. When you go through rivers of difficulty, you will not drown! When you walk through the fire of oppression, you will not be burned up–the flames will not consume you. For I am the Lord your God."

(Isaiah 43:2-3)

I had two options when I found out about Giana's diagnosis. Either I could find someone to blame for it or ask Jesus to comfort me in these challenges. I chose the latter and can gladly say it was the right thing to do. Even after it has been so long since the whole ordeal, I will never regret choosing God over anything else.

Events like this only teach you that no matter how complicated your life gets, you must never give up and keep seeking God's light to help you in grim, troublesome times.

Anthony was, for the most part, enjoying normal activities and sports. He tried inline skating, soccer, snowboarding, riding an ATV, and ice hockey, to name a few. One day, when Anthony was in 6th grade, the school contacted me regarding some chest pain that he was experiencing. At first, it was written off as heartburn, and the school nurse had given him some acid reflux medication. Then, I received two more phone calls from Anthony, indicating he had severe chest pain. I knew Anthony had a very high tolerance for pain, so this was not to be taken lightly. I arrived at his school and took him to a local emergency room.

The ER doctor was worried it was something with Anthony's heart, so he referred us to a pediatric cardiologist. Upon examination and testing, it was revealed that Anthony had a spontaneous pneumothorax (collapsed lung). This may have been due to a snowboarding accident approximately one week earlier. I rode in an ambulance with Anthony to Children's Hospital in Pittsburgh, where Anthony had a chest tube inserted and was treated without any complications. Wow, that was another scary event, and God once again faithfully guided us through the rough waters.

"The Lord will keep you from all harm—He will watch over your life; the Lord will watch over your coming and going both now and forevermore."

(Psalm 121:7-8)

"Thou art my hiding place; Thou dost preserve me from trouble; Thou dost surround me with songs of deliverance."

(Psalm 32:7)

Chapter 10: Accident Aftermath

*HOPE Rx "But as for me, I watch in **HOPE** for the Lord, I wait for God my Savior; my God will hear me."*

(Micah 7:7)

Feeding my children an organic diet drove their inner curiosity to explore their pathways in life. My constant efforts encouraged them to eat a balanced diet full of nourishment.

Anthony became a raw food vegan in his teens and used to forage for wild foods in the woods. He had long hair and was very lean and athletic. He often used to walk in the woods barefoot, grounding with the earth and climbing trees, so he earned the nickname *Tarzan*.

He also had an herbalist mentor who helped him adapt to this lifestyle; soon, he became more passionate about following natural and healthy regimes. He became quite passionate about raw foods, and he built a website called "The Wild Alchemist" and started his blog. Within a short time, he gained thousands of followers. People were impressed and admired his lifestyle choices at such a young age.

Anthony even went to Boulder, Colorado, to study at the North American Institute for Medical Herbalism. My son inspired many of his friends and colleagues about natural health and well-being. He also obtained a nutritional certification and did some local public speaking, as he was a big advocate of superfoods.

Anthony planted trays full of wheatgrass, and we purchased a wheatgrass juice extractor. He made herbal tinctures and brewed medicinal mushrooms in a crockpot. We rented office space from a naturopathic doctor to give Anthony opportunities to help other people, and he did.

Our family flourished and kept busy with school activities, sports events, music lessons, and family vacations for a good ten-year stretch or so without any major adverse health events. We made lots of memories and shared many beautiful moments together. Things were pretty normal and much less stressful through that period of time. The children seemed to embrace their youth and were enjoying life, traveling, and expanding their horizons.

In October 2021, Ginelle and I planned to accompany Anthony to Nashville, Tennessee, to celebrate his 31st birthday. Together, we attended a complementary alternative cancer conference, where we had an amazing experience building links with many of Anthony's well-known natural health and wellness warriors. We made many unforgettable memories that weekend, and I was so happy to bring Anthony to this event. Seeing him grow up with his siblings was so gratifying to our family and such a blessing.

Anthony also learned different experiences with so much resilience. He found a passion for a natural lifestyle, and I couldn't have been more thankful to Jesus. He made this all happen by turning all the impossibilities into possibilities until one fateful day.

It was November 15, 2021. I was the only family member in Erie during that time when I got an unexpected call from the emergency room of a local hospital stating, "Ma'am, your son, Anthony, has been in a motor vehicle accident."

Before that happened, I was trying to get on the phone with him because he was supposed to come to our house after his class that evening. Only after the hospital call did I realize why he wasn't responding to my calls and messages.

As soon as I got the call from the hospital, I left everything I was doing and rushed to him. As I was driving to the emergency room, there were trucks, ambulances, and police on another road that was closed off. I immediately prayed for that person's life safety, knowing that my own son's life was at stake.

I was in such a hurry, and little did I realize that the dreadful scene was my own precious son's car accident.

When I arrived at the hospital ER, the first thing I saw was Anthony's sweatpants, which were full of blood and all torn up. His condition was serious and needed to be taken care of immediately. Both of his femurs had been fractured during the catastrophic accident. The doctors took him to the operating room urgently for surgery. While I was there, I was shaking in fear and disbelief. I continuously prayed to God for his recovery.

This whole scenario brought up so many awful and traumatic memories of my brother and father's accident in 1985. I was lost in thoughts, and being alone at that moment was killing me from the inside. I wanted someone by my side and needed a shoulder to cry on. So, I called my good Christian friend and coworker at the hospital to wait with me while Anthony was in the operating room for his surgery.

I could not understand how it all happened. I couldn't even recognize his car when I went to the junkyard to see it. There was busted-up glass and a smashed vehicle in an atrocious condition, not even resembling a car whatsoever. All I could think was that God was not done with my son and allowed him to survive such an ordeal for a reason.

It was clear that God had more plans for my son and wanted him to live his life to the fullest. The police officer said Anthony's Honda Civic and a semi-truck collided head-on. Anthony was trapped in the vehicle for one hour before being rescued. He had a total of ten fractures from the waist down. It was a miracle that he survived such a horrendous accident without being paralyzed.

Anthony sustained a severe concussion as well, and his left ear suffered hearing impairment for some time—blood kept oozing out of that ear.

After his initial surgery, Anthony's other femur was operated on after a two-week break due to being a more complex fracture. He developed a blood clot in that leg after the surgery.

Once that was over, he spent two months in the trauma center. I spent every single day with him at the hospital, giving him juices, smoothies, supplements, herbal tinctures, and teas to speed up his recovery.

We listened to many inspirational songs and devotionals and grew stronger through these moments of suffering. After two months in the trauma unit, Anthony was transferred to a rehabilitation hospital for two more months. I came across a song by Taurence Wells that really ministered to my soul called "God's Not Done with You."

Standing in your ruins feels a lot like the end

So used to losing, you're afraid to try again

Right now all you see are ashes where there was a flame

Truth is that you're not forgotten

'Cause Grace knows your name

God's not done with you

Even with your broken heart and your wounds and your scars

God's not done with you

Even when you're lost and it's hard and you're falling apart

God's not done with you

It's not over, it's only begun

So don't hide don't run

'Cause God's not done with you

There's a light you don't notice

Until you're standing in the dark

And there's a strength that's growing

Inside your shattered heart

He's got a plan, this is part of it

He's gonna finish what He started

He's got a plan this is part of it

He's gonna finish what He started

God's not done with you

He's not done

God's not done with you

No, He's not done

God's not done with you.

We were once again at the same place where we started; trauma bonded at the hospital together day in and day out.

We were indeed traumatized and quite broken at this point because this was another calamity we were facing together as a family. Sometimes, I wonder:

Why can't I beat these fiery trials?

Why has God chosen me for these misfortunes?

But I know the answer. I think it's because of my strong faith in Him; He has chosen me for this trial because He knows I can handle this. God has always provided me with grace, and now I have accepted that His way is always the best way.

"Satan cannot test us beyond God's will. All adversity is sifted through the permissive will of God and has a divine

purpose. It is not meant to sink us but to sanctify us. It is not meant to hinder us but to help us."

(Charles Stanley)

*"I wait for the Lord, my whole being waits, and in His word I put my **HOPE**." **(Psalm 130:5)***

Chapter 11: Safe Storms

HOPE Rx *"The Lord taketh pleasure in them that fear Him, in those that **HOPE** in His mercy."*

(Psalm 147:11)

"Save me, O God; For the waters are come in unto my soul. I sink in deep mire, where there is no standing: I am come into deep waters, where the floods overflow me. I am weary of my crying: my throat is dried. Mine eyes fail while I wait for my God."

(Psalms 69:1-3)

Our lives on Earth, at times, are so woven into pain and suffering that we forget the good moments.

When we face constant hardships in life, we often believe there is no end. Sometimes, unexpected suffering seizes us in a way that we cannot define, and that pain impacts us physically, emotionally, relationally, and spiritually.

Life doesn't spare any of us from experiencing storm-like hurdles. They often have varying intensities, durations, and frequencies. We must realize that when the storm rages, only Jesus can bring real **HOPE** and good news in the midst of it.

We have to trust in His power and presence, even though there are howling winds, high seas, and unknown territory. God is bigger than whatever storm we come across. His existence is bound to comfort us and quiet our fears.

It is imperative to hold tightly to the One navigating through the storms because only He can calm them. I have been a part of these storms most of my life and feel pity for those who face similar trials. We might feel that suffering may sometimes be undeserved, but it is never purposeless. It comes for our good and His glory. We should learn to trust and obey God because there is no other way.

"My ears had heard of you, but now my eyes have seen you. Therefore, I despise myself and repent in dust and ashes."

(Job 42:5-6)

There is no storm without a cause, just like no difficulty without a solution. These trials are preparing us for eternity. God is always there to rescue his people from their sorrows.

"For our light and momentary troubles are achieving for us an eternal glory that far outweighs them all."

(2 Corinthians 4:17)

There are always good and bad times in the storms of life, but trusting in God's power through the dark tunnels requires deep faith. The tunnel of my life was long, challenging, and uncertain. It was often flooded with fear, stress, anxiety, exhaustion, sleepless nights, and difficult medical decisions.

We must believe that our grief will end and that none of it will be wasted. It will bear fruit for us and others if we let it. Our real enemy is not that which kills the body but rather that which kills the soul.

"Who shall separate us from the love of Christ? Shall trouble or hardship or persecution or famine or nakedness or danger or sword? No, in all these things, we are more than conquerors through Him who loved us."

(Romans 8:35, 37)

During all these times, I felt helpless but not **HOPE**LESS. God gave me many signs and confirmations that He was with me throughout those times. These are the lessons I learned:

1. Life is very short and fragile. You should enjoy each day to the fullest and take one day at a time. Don't overburden yourself with thoughts that you have no control over.

2. Caring is a form of language that removes barriers and strengthens the bond. At times, it was very hard to feel God's love and presence, but it became obvious through other caring Christians and fellow believers.

3. We can try our best to save our children, but remember that we are only stewards of them; they belong to God.

4. There are often times when we seem to be totally out of control, but that's when God is totally in control. We must yield to His divine authority and rejoice in His sovereignty.

5. God foreknows the trials we will face in our lifetime. He promises us His presence, comfort, strength, mercy, and grace to endure them victoriously.

*"God's delays are not **God's** denials."*

(Dr. James Dobson)

6. God is able to do the impossible, and human calculations have no place with God.

"For with God, nothing shall be impossible."

(Luke 1:37)

7. We all know that eventually, life becomes easier, just like rainbows follow the rain; light overpowers darkness; thorns turn into flowers; crosses turn into crowns; tribulations become triumphs; messes become messages; and tests become testimonies.

8. As long as there is life, there is **HOPE**.

"You should trust God independent of your understanding of the circumstances."

(Dr. James Dobson)

9. You need to decide and choose a side in life. You can either have dependence on God or despair and become better or bitter.

10. Read the book of Psalms and stick to the word for encouragement and truths.

"Wait on the Lord: Be of good courage, and He shall strengthen thine heart: wait, I say, on the Lord."

(Psalm 27:14)

11. Prayer and fasting alter things and make a difference. You should believe that miracles are real. *(Anthony is definitely one of them)*

12. Keep a Journal through the trials so you can periodically look back and reflect on God's faithfulness with tears of thankfulness. My pastor said that faith looks behind, **HOPE** looks ahead, and love looks both ways.

13. Fight adversity with faith. The best test of faith is when it is exercised. Faith is like a muscle; the more it's exercised, the bigger and stronger it gets.

"God may not always take away your trials, but He will prepare you and take you through. His provisions include His presence, protection, a pathway, and peace."

(Charles Stanley)

We are never alone in the race of life. It is said that,

"If God takes you to it, He will get you through it."

"Trials provide a potential for spiritual growth and understanding of God. God's mountains of difficulty are His stepping stones."

(Mrs. Charles Cowman)

These points are the excerpts of all the experiences I had, whether good or bad. I went through times when I had no clue what tomorrow would bring. However, God held my hand and helped me through the storms. He blessed Anthony with a new life despite all the contradictions from the doctors that he would not make it.

My son is a grown-up man, now 34-years-old. He is living a healthy life, and God-willing will be able to pursue his passion. Although his life journey was not like that of an ordinary child, he managed to escape the darkness and shine bright. His attitude on life is indescribable. He has no bitterness and holds no grudges. He is an absolute light to our family, and we admire his bravery and courage. Anthony's nickname changed from *"Tarzan"* to *"Rocky"* and *"The Comeback Kid."*

The only thing we have been given control over is the authority to do the best we can. This should be seen as a positive thing despite all the negativity. God has the power to turn all the tables, but the only thing that we can do is **HOPE** for His mercy and blessings. Our belief in God's power makes things possible.

"To appoint unto them that mourn in Zion, to give unto them beauty for ashes, the oil of joy for mourning, the garment of praise for the spirit of heaviness; that they might be called trees of righteousness, the planting of the Lord, that He might be glorified."

(Isaiah 61:3)

The promises of God's word allow us to see the best in any situation and help us keep a positive outlook.

A song by Douglas Miller (songwriter Florence B Price) that resonates so well with me is called "My Soul Has Been Anchored in the Lord" and it says:

Though the storms keep on raging in my life

And sometimes it's hard to tell the night from day

*Still that **HOPE** that lies within is reassured*

As I keep my eyes upon the distant shore

I know He'll lead me safely to that blessed place He has prepared

But if the storms don't cease

And if the winds keep on blowing

My soul has been anchored in the Lord

Oh, I realize that sometimes in this life, we're gonna be tossed

By the waves and the currents that seem so fierce

But in the Word of God, I've got an anchor

And it keeps me steadfast and unmovable

Despite the tides

But if the storms don't cease

And just in case the winds, they keep on blowing in my life

My soul's been anchored in the Lord

The pillars may roll, the breakers may dash

I shall not sway because He holds me fast

So dark the day, clouds in the sky

I know it's alright, 'cause Jesus is mine

(Psalm 34:19-20) Many are the afflictions of the righteous: But the Lord delivereth him out of them all. He keepeth all his bones: Not one of them is broken.

Chapter 12: Hopeful Healing

Try to imagine the overwhelming shock of a diagnosis that your child has a life-threatening terminal illness. These words pierce your heart as you begin to wonder how you will ever get through a parent's worst nightmare. It's like not knowing whether or not you will ever hit the finish line of this marathon with a positive outcome of winning the race. Sometimes, trials seem to have no expiration date. Regardless of the trials we have faced, are facing, or will soon face, we are called to run our race with every bit of stamina we have.

(I Cor 9:24) *"Know ye not that they which run in a race run all, but once receiveth the prize? So run, that ye may obtain."*

Pain and suffering are woven into our lives on earth, like the sudden onslaught of pain, grief, and loss that engulfed my family multiple times. Sometimes, we feel like God abandons us in our afflictions, and God who permits them finds our hearts stricken with a paralyzing fear. We can lose the firm footing from which to climb out of the abyss of our pain and wonder why the God of comfort would allow such torment.

It is comforting to know we never have to face pain alone and that nothing can separate us from the love of God. **(Romans 8:38-39)** states, *"For I am convinced that neither death nor life, neither angels nor demons, neither the present* *nor the future, nor any powers, neither height nor depth nor anything else in all creation, will be able to separate us from the love of God that is in Christ Jesus our Lord."* Pain may be part of the story, but it's not the end of the story. **(Job 23:10):** *"But He knoweth the way that I take: when He hath tried me, I shall come forth as gold."*

God uses everything we've been through to bring out the very best in us. He will get the glory from our life.

You may be in a season of suffering and struggle. God will restore and bring you out better. He turns our mourning into dancing, our sorrow into joy, and our weeping into laughter. **(Psalm 30:11-12)** *"You have turned my mourning into dancing."* God has the final say, and He not only controls our lives but also our circumstances. Our pain has a purpose, and God has plans to use this pain for His good and glory. "Weeping may endure for night, but joy cometh in the morning." **(Psalm 30:5)**

We are to speak what we seek and call things that are not as though they are. **(Romans 4:17)** tells us, *"God, who quickeneth the dead, and calleth those things which be not as though they were."* This means that God speaks the end result. We are called to believe and receive God's promises.

"In thee, O LORD, do I put my trust: let me never be put to confusion. Deliver me in thy righteousness, and cause me to escape: incline thine ear unto me, and save me. Be thou my strong habitation, whereunto I may continually resort: thou hast given commandment to save me; for thou art my rock and my fortress. Deliver me, O my God, out of the

*hand of the wicked, out of the hand of the unrighteous and cruel man. For thou art my **HOPE**, O Lord GOD: thou art my trust from my youth. By thee have I been holden up from the womb: thou art he that took me out of my mother's bowels: my praise shall be continually of thee. I am as a wonder unto many; but thou art my strong refuge. Let my mouth be filled with thy praise and with thy honor all the day. Cast me not off in the time of old age; forsake me not when my strength faileth."*

(Psalm 71:1-7)

During our difficult years, I fed myself with Bible promises from the Book of Psalms because it provided the consolation I desperately needed. Regardless of what life was going to bring our way, God had a plan filled with **HOPE** as long as we believed that God is who He says He is and that He would do what He said He would do. It became clear that God used my pain to help others through cancer, so consequently, I became a cancer coach with tremendous empathy for others. Redemptive pain is the highest and ultimate use of our pain. Knowing that Jesus is with us will strengthen our faith and bring us peace.

It is crucial to spend time in a resting and hiding place where our hearts and minds can be restored and strengthened from all the struggles and challenges in life. This is where we find the all-sufficiency of God and are able to leave with a renewed courage to face each day. God, in His infinite goodness and sovereignty, is in control even when we don't understand the reasons for suffering. The opposite of **HOPE** is dread, which Satan uses to keep us from trusting in God. Instead of dread, our family had to believe that good things would be ahead. We had to choose whether to live in dread or in **HOPE**, but we knew we could not do both at the same time. **HOPE** is a favorable and confident expectation. It is an expectant attitude that something good is going to happen and that things will work out no matter what situation we are facing. Holding on to our confidence in God's power, especially when our circumstances defy our understanding, can lift our hardships to something higher and of worth because He is always there. God does not waste any of our tears, and these dark seasons are tools He uses to mold and shape us into who He desires.

I pray **(Eph 3:16)** over you *"that He would grant you, according to the riches of His glory, to be strengthened with might by His Spirit in the inner man;"* **(Eph 3:11-13)** *according to the eternal purpose which He purposed in Christ Jesus our Lord: in whom we have boldness and access with confidence by the faith of Him. Wherefore I desire that ye faint not at my tribulations for you, which is your glory."* We can have boldness, confidence, and great expectations, even when our battles look hopeless. We must learn to restore our confidence in God and trust Him by focusing on His goodness, not our circumstances. **(Eph 3:20)** says, *"Now unto Him that is able to do exceedingly abundantly above all that we ask or think, according to the power that worketh in us. Unto Him be glory in the church by Christ Jesus throughout all ages, world without end."*

(Matt 28:20): *"Lo, I am with you always, even unto the end of the world."* Using the example of Paul in the Bible, he was burdened to the point of despairing life itself, but he learned that this happened so that he would learn to rely on God rather than himself. How we respond to desperate times tells a lot about our character. Having an expectant **HOPE** is an anchor of the soul. **(Psalm 39:7):** *"And now, Lord, what wait I for? My **HOPE** is in thee."*

God's grace, protection, and provision are sources of **HOPE** that we cannot fully comprehend until we experience them amidst circumstances that try to destroy us. Paul said in **(II Corinthians 4:8-9)** *"We are afflicted in every way, but not crushed; perplexed but not despairing; persecuted, but not forsaken; struck down, but not destroyed."* Never forget God's love and faithful presence and persevere confidently, expecting that we are not alone or forgotten.

A song called "Stand" by Donnie McClurkin says:

What do you do when you've done all you can

And it seems like it's never enough

And what do you say when your friends turn away

And you're all alone

Tell me what do you give when you've given your all

And it seems like you can't make it through

Well you just stand, when there's nothing left to do

You just stand, watch the Lord see you through

Yes after you've done all you can, you just stand

Tell me how do you handle the guilt of your past

Tell me how do you deal with the shame

And how can you smile while your heart has been broken

And filled with pain filled with pain

Tell me what do you give when you've given your all

And it seems like you can't make it through

Child you just stand when there's nothing left to do

You just stand watch the Lord see you through

Yes after you've done all you can, you just stand

Stand and be sure

Be not entangled in that bondage again, you just stand and endure

For God has a purpose yes God has a plan, tell me

What do you do when you've done all you can

And it seems like you can't make it through

Child you just stand

Don't your dare give up

Through the storm stand

Stand through the rain

Through the hurt stand

Yeah through the pain you

Don't you bow (stand) and don't you bend (stand)

Don't give up (stand) no don't give in (you just)

Hold on (stand), just be strong (stand)

God will step in (stand), it won't be long no (you just stand)

After you've done all you can
After you've gone through the hurt
After you've gone through the pain
After you've gone through the storm
After you've gone through the rain
After you've done all you can
You just stand

Chapter 13: Revelatory Reflections

HOPE Rx *"Therefore being justified by faith, we have peace with God through our Lord Jesus Christ: by whom also we have access by faith into this grace wherein we stand, and rejoice in **HOPE** of the glory of God."*

(Rom 5:1-2)

I repetitively asked myself,

"Were there any benefits to going through so many fiery trials?"

I had lost my dad and brother tragically at a young age and, later in life, my precious mom in 2020. Anthony battled cancer twice and had as many surgeries as birthdays; Giana had meningitis as a baby; Victor had a rare platelet disorder as a baby; Anthony almost died in a barn fire in 5th grade and had a collapsed lung at school in 6th grade. He also had a snowboarding and an ATV accident. Anthony even suffered a seizure in the hospital and ended up in the ICU multiple times throughout his lifetime. I had a total of three miscarriages and came very close to losing Anthony in a near-fatal motor vehicle accident. It just looked like it was never going to end, but with each passing moment, I grew stronger and developed an endurance I never knew I had.

"No unbelief made him waver concerning the promise of God, but he grew strong in his faith as he gave glory to God, fully convinced that God was able to do what he had promised."

(Romans 4:20–21)

After facing so many losses and near losses in life, I developed a heightened sensitivity for others going through tough times and health challenges. It was because God equipped me to understand and comfort others. There were times when things were happening so fast that I didn't have the time or opportunity to process them; they were one after another. During those times, I sought help through books, music, and videos, which included the following resources:

- John Hagee Healing Scripture tapes

- Charles Stanley's teachings included (Storms of Life, Advancing Through Adversity, Keeping the Faith, and The Believer's Valley Experiences)

- Dr. James Dobson (When God Doesn't Make Sense)

- Diane M Komp (Hope Springs from Mended Places: Images of Grace in the Shadows of Life)

- Kay Arthur (Where are you, Lord, when Bad Things Happen?)

- Mrs. Charles E. Cowman (Springs in the Valley/Streams in the Desert)

- Daily Light on the Daily Path Devotional

Some of the songs that kept me encouraged and inspired during those times were;

- Jesus' Rocking Chair (The Greenes)

- I'm Still Here (Bruce Carroll)

- Through It All (Andrae Crouch)

I used to sing these lyrics repeatedly.

"I've had many tears and sorrows

I've had questions for tomorrow

There's been times I didn't know right from wrong

But in every situation

God gave me blessed consolation

That my trials come to only make me strong

Through it all

Through it all

I've learned to trust in Jesus

I've learned to trust in God

Through it all

Through it all

I've learned to depend upon His Word

I've been to lots of places

I've seen a lot of faces

There's been times I felt so all alone

But in my lonely hours

Yes, those precious lonely hours

Jesus lets me know that I was His own

Through it all

Through it all

I've learned to trust in Jesus

I've learned to trust in God."

I learned that everyone is suffering uniquely in their own way. We all measure it differently because it is all relative. We, as humans, try our best to wrestle and win the fight against the calamities. These devastating feelings build many questions in our heads.

"Why does God allow his people to suffer?

Why does God allow such torment?

Why doesn't God love me?

Why doesn't God take the pain away from me?"

This sense of injustice is augmented when the innocent and young ones suffer, especially when it's your own precious child. The grief of our little ones seems so undeserved that it makes our hearts ache. But as believers, we know it is never without purpose. God tests the faith of His people by giving them multiple challenges. The Lord allows us to experience these circumstances that drain our lives and display our weakness right when strength is needed the most. Job discovered that even without the answers and relief from suffering, He had all he needed in God.

"I know that you can do all things; no purpose of yours can be thwarted."

(Job 42:1-6)

The lesson learned from Job's story is to keep your belief in God despite unanswered questions and gain true knowledge of the cross as God's answer to misery. Job faced catastrophes in his life, one after another. But he kept his faith in God intact, which helped him navigate the storms.

I could easily relate my life circumstances to Job's, so far out at sea in life-threatening storms with no familiar landmarks in sight. Job knew that the storm was highly intense, but he kept all his energy and focused solely on how big God was and not the size of the storm. He praised the Lord even while bearing pain—a definite example of perseverance and a sacrifice of praise.

My family recovered from the storms because of God's grace and mercy. We just fixed our compass in the right direction that permitted us to hold ourselves as each crisis showed up to deepen our relationship with Him. God's power and wisdom are infinitely beyond our imagination. The solution to misery is found in learning to rest in God's grace and to trust in His power.

"God whispers to us in our pleasures, speaks to us in our conscience, and shouts to us in our pain."

(CS Lewis)

Have you ever wondered why evil usually prospers while good ones are tested repeatedly?

Why do bad people seem to benefit while good people seem to struggle and encounter difficulty?

Life didn't always seem fair when, despite my countless efforts to treat Anthony's cancer, it recurred. Why did one human being have to go through so much at such a young age?

"For I was envious of the arrogant as I saw the prosperity of the wicked."

(Psalm 73: 2)

We get a clear understanding of life events when we look at them from the rearview mirror. If I look back on my story, there was uncertainty, doubts, pain, and despair.

There was a time when I had lost **HOPE** and didn't know what else to do.

But God helped me to get back on my feet when I sought refuge in the holy book of the Bible. It is mandatory to spend solitude in God's remembrance to strengthen your soul, heart, and mind. We must learn to restore our confidence in God and trust the process in His goodness, not our circumstances. This is something we all need to work on.

"I am with you always, even to the end of the age."

(Matt 28:20)

The human mind is unable to comprehend the mysteries behind God's plan. In that case, we should keep our confidence in God's power, especially when our circumstances defy our understanding. God's power, in abundance, will then lift our hardships and bless us with something of worth because He is always there to help His people. You should know that these dark times are the tools God uses to mold and shape us into stronger people.

(**I Thess 5:11**) *"Wherefore comfort yourselves together, and edify one another, even as also ye do."*

I truly believe God called me to write this book and share my family's experiences to edify, motivate, and inspire you in difficult situations. Our story shows how getting through the same experiences with a sense of **HOPE** is possible. I desire you to overcome your fears now that you've heard how our family traveled the same roads. God will cause grace to abound, and He will fuel you and refresh you. We are all human, and all of us experience weariness of heart. Remember, God is with you, strengthens you, and upholds you with His righteous right hand. He will help you walk by faith when nothing seems to make sense, and no matter how tired you feel, keep on seeking God for His infinite wisdom and ask Him for supernatural strength. **HOPE** truly is the most potent medicine and the prescription needed to mitigate the adverse side effects of fear, worry, doubt, and hopelessness.

HOPE can help you break through your barriers.

"Blessed be God, even the Father of our Lord Jesus Christ, the Father of mercies, and the God of all comfort; who comforteth us in all our tribulation, that we may be able to comfort them which are in any trouble, by the comfort wherewith we ourselves are comforted of God."

(2 Cor 1:3-4)

HOPE and *faith* oftentimes go hand in hand. **HOPE** gave us the strength to endure so many hardships and long waiting periods. God used our trying times to help develop our character and endurance.

Ultimately, we must accept that God's plan is infinitely better than our own could ever be, and our childlike faith, belief, and **HOPE** in God catches us each and every time we fall.

(Psalm 66:10-12) *"For thou, O God hast proved us: Thou hast tried us, as silver is tried. Thou broughtest us into the net; Thou laidst affliction upon our loins. Thou hast caused men to ride over our heads; We went through fire and through water: But thou broughtest us out into a wealthy place."*

A final reflection on a song by Abby and Chris Eaton called "Hope in the Darkness."

You are God's own

His joy, His song His treasure

Created in His likeness

A light that burns forever

You are God's own

Safe, secure, protected

Through every trial and terror

His love will hold you tight forever

Who can know the pain you are carrying?

Who can even begin to understand?

There is HOPE in the darkness
For the God of love is always by your side
Just hold on, He is faithful
He will pierce the veil and fill your heart with light
There is HOPE in the darkness
You are God's own
He knows you and He loves you
He goes behind you and before you
He guides your every step
Draw near to Him
With a heart of worship
Make it a holy place where darkness cannot live
You can know the comfort of belonging
You can rise upon the wings of peace
There is HOPE in the darkness
For the God of love is always by your side
Just hold on, He is faithful
He will pierce the veil and fill your heart with light
There is HOPE, there is HOPE, there is HOPE, so
Have the faith to lean on the sovereignty of God
Sing a song of worship even when the cause seems lost
Bring your imperfections, bring your heartache and your
pain
To the God of mercy who will wipe your tears away
There is HOPE in the darkness
For the God of love is always by your side

Just hold on, He is faithful
He will pierce the veil and fill your heart with light
There is HOPE, there is HOPE
There is HOPE in the darkness

As I stumbled across another song called HOPE in the Darkness by Merry Lee she sings…

When the night seems so long
And the darkness surrounds me strong
I lift my eyes up to you and find HOPE in your truth
You are my HOPE in the darkness
Shining light on the path before me
You will guide me through this storm
Oh Lord you are my HOPE
Hallelujah

As for my husband Tony and I, it's been 35 years of courageous commitment through…

Trials and triumphs
Devastating diagnoses
Hardships and healing
Miracles and the mundane
Blessings and burdens
Victories and ventures

Through the joys and through the pain, our faithful love, strength, compassion, and devotion have remained.

God's plan is greater than our pain. You will find your purpose in your pain. His love transforms our hurt into **HOPE.** Trust in His purpose and find strength in His promises. This is the **HOPE** prescription...

Hold

Onto God's

Promises

Everyday

www.ingramcontent.com/pod-product-compliance
Lightning Source LLC
Chambersburg PA
CBHW071335150726
47997CB00002B/738